PEACE, POWER,

and a

SOUND MIND

An Emerging Approach in the
Treatment of Addictions

Rhonda S. McBride, PhD, LCDC

BALBOA.
PRESS
A DIVISION OF HAY HOUSE

Balboa Press books may be ordered through booksellers or by contacting:

Balboa Press
A Division of Hay House
1663 Liberty Drive
Bloomington, IN 47403
www.balboapress.com
1-(877) 407-4847

Because of the dynamic nature of the Internet, any web addresses or links contained in this book may have changed since publication and may no longer be valid. The views expressed in this work are solely those of the author and do not necessarily reflect the views of the publisher, and the publisher hereby disclaims any responsibility for them.

The author of this book does not dispense medical advice or prescribe the use of any technique as a form of treatment for physical, emotional, or medical problems without the advice of a physician, either directly or indirectly. The intent of the author is only to offer information of a general nature to help you in your quest for emotional and spiritual well-being. In the event you use any of the information in this book for yourself, which is your constitutional right, the author and the publisher assume no responsibility for your actions.

Any people depicted in stock imagery provided by Thinkstock are models, and such images are being used for illustrative purposes only.
Certain stock imagery © Thinkstock.

ISBN: 978-1-4525-4044-3 (e)
ISBN: 978-1-4525-4043-6 (sc)
ISBN: 978-1-4525-4042-9 (hc)

Library of Congress Control Number: 2011918402

Printed in the United States of America

Balboa Press rev. date: 11/02/2011

This book is dedicated to the many clients along the way who have shared their stories, deepest feelings, and their incredible courage with me.

Contents

Prologue

This book was born from a deep sense of gratitude to the amazing people along the way who lovingly and persistently held up a mirror in front of me, showing me my value, strength, and ability—even when I could not see it myself. As a clinician primarily concerned with addictions, as well as emotional issues including anger, depression, and anxiety, it has long been my goal to create a program that would give clients tools for healing and personal growth, one that would reach beyond the Twelve Steps of Alcoholics Anonymous (AA) to address all aspects of people's lives. In January 2000, I took the first step on this journey when I opened A New Approach Counseling Services. This practice encompasses individual and group counseling for those who do not necessarily need or seek a higher level of care, or who are perhaps uncomfortable with treatment that teaches that AA is the only way to obtain sobriety. I took the second step in realizing my vision in 2005, when I became an affiliate of The Right Step, offering an intensive substance abuse outpatient program for adolescents and adults. Drawing upon my strong belief in holistic health, and my understanding of the healing power of AA's Twelve Steps, I created a program that merged the two modalities. The acceptance by the community and the clinical outcome of this program has been tremendous. Throughout, my objective has been to empower addicts with the coping skills necessary to find balance in all areas of their lives. The approach I outline in this book accomplishes that objective.

My journey in exploring healing modalities has been both a personal and professional one. Therefore, I will begin by explaining my sometimes arduous journey from 1995 to the present (although, as we all know, our stories encompass all of our life experiences and lessons).

After several years of marriage and a difficult and bitter divorce, I found myself alone, confused, and deeply angry. This anger, stemming from a sense of loss and survival, became a driving force for me. It pushed me through the process of grief, through the insanity of an addiction to alcohol and toxic relationships, through deep self-exploration, and finally to a place of personal empowerment and acceptance of myself.

During my marriage, my husband decided that we should return to the religion of his childhood. Not knowing quite what to expect. and desperately wanting my marriage to work, I agreed to follow along. Having grown up in a fairly liberal, open-minded church, what followed was completely outside my realm of understanding. We began keeping the Sabbath from sundown Friday to sundown Saturday. We did not attend a formal church; rather,, we participated in home church services with other like-minded folks. Our children did not go to public schools; instead, I homeschooled them. Doctors and traditional medicine were forbidden. There were dietary restrictions and a host of thou-shalt-nots. Religion, which had always been a source of comfort and peace for me, became a source of argument, contention, and fear. Whenever any of us would step out of line, the Bible was brought out for instruction and reproof.

This web of propriety hid a dark side: one of anger, control, and domination. Men were definitely considered the more important gender. At times, I thought I would lose my mind. I certainly lost my sense of self. Terrified of being alone and with no idea of how I would support my children and myself, I stayed and tried to make our lives as peaceful and normal as possible.

It was not all bad. I loved homeschooling my children. Everything became a learning experience. We lived in the country, where we raised chickens and goats and grew vegetables. We lived very simply. I believe this experience fortified us for what was to come.

Out of consideration for my children, I will not go into the details of the deeply traumatic event that led to my divorce, as it does not alter the focus of this work. But it was enough to shake the very foundation of our belief system. In the depths of depression, feeling totally lost, I moved home with my three children to my parents' house. My daughter was just beginning high school, and my two sons were in the first and fifth grades. Although they were academically prepared, entering public school was a social and emotional adjustment for them.

One morning, over coffee, I told my dad that I needed to go to college and take a computer course or something. I had not worked in many years, and I knew that I had to figure out a way to support my children and give them a sense of normalcy again—whatever normal was.

On the way to the local college, I had a major panic attack. Everything began spinning and I couldn't breathe. I pulled the car over and began crying deeply and uncontrollably. I cried from the depths of my soul. I began yelling at God and telling him that I was furious with him. If he were so damned all-powerful, how had I ended up in this situation? Why hadn't he intervened and protected my family? We had, after all, been faithful to all the rules, expectations, and dogmas, only to end up afraid, lonely, and broke. At that point, I told God that he could just go screw himself.

As I calmed down, I sat there, waiting for lightning to strike or something after my disrespectful tirade. Instead, I began to experience a deep sense of peace unlike anything I had ever felt before. Somehow, I knew that God understood and could handle my anger. I didn't know how, but I knew everything would be okay.

I went home and talked this over with my mother. I cried a bit more and told her that I was afraid that God had abandoned me and that I was losing my mind. She informed me firmly but lovingly that God had not abandoned me; that he had, in fact, led me out of the darkness, and that losing my mind was simply not an option. I think I was angry at her, too, at that point. I thought that if I lost my mind, maybe I could just escape the pain and fear, and everything would be easier. But, I also understood that all my anger and bitterness were keeping me from being there for my children emotionally. I went into my room, opened my Bible, and told God that, after reading this book for many years, it no longer made sense to me. I had to wipe the slate clean and start the journey to God all over again. I felt a glimmer of peace.

The next day, I tried again to go to college and at least ask some questions. I spoke to a counselor and went to the financial aid office.

Before the day was over, I had enrolled for fifteen credit hours, applied for financial aid, and even gotten a job in the financial aid office!

My first field of study was criminal justice. I was still angry and looking for justification. But, I quickly realized this was not the path for me, and switched my major to human services. I wanted to understand what my children were going through and how to help them. I loved the coursework and the people. There were many times I left school in tears as I learned about family dynamics and the long-term effects of an abusive marriage and divorce. The process also forced me to look at my own childhood issues and how those experiences affected my decisions as an adult.

Studying for years to become a psychologist was financially impossible, so I began studies in chemical dependency. This major allowed me to make a living while continuing my education. After the first few semesters, I began working at the Cypress-Fairbanks school district's Alternative Learning Center while completing my internship.

While working at the Alternative Learning Center I met a woman named Nancy Rose. Nancy was my supervisor and mentor. She put me in the classroom and told me to combine my instincts as a mother with my creativity and skills as a counselor, and everything else would turn out right. Almost all of my students were there because of drug and alcohol issues. Many had serious legal issues, and many had devastating home lives. I'd never dreamed I would work in a public school, especially this one! I loved working with the kids. I connected with them and felt a sense of purpose.

Meanwhile, my children were adjusting to public school and life in a new and different environment. My parents went from having an empty nest for several years to having a brood at home again. There were many challenges for all of us. Without the love and support of my mom and dad, this journey would have been much more difficult, and I am eternally grateful for our time together.

Desperately wanting to be loved and accepted, I began dating. I ended up with a series of toxic relationships. It seemed I was addicted to men who were alcoholic and controlling. I began drinking, too, and my drinking led to many compromising and painful situations.

Although I was great at my job, my personal life suffered. After a whirlwind romance, I ended up marrying a police officer who had a background as a detective working with abuse cases. He seemed so understanding and kind. I enjoyed the "protection" he offered as well. However, shortly into the marriage, he became extremely controlling and abusive. This affected my relationship with my children, and I became extremely depressed. My self-esteem was nearly nonexistent. After a year-and-a-half, I came home from work one night and found my husband drunk, angry, and violent. From deep inside, I found the strength to end the relationship.

I began attending Twelve Step meetings and gained an understanding of the depths of my addictions, both to toxic relationships and to alcohol. I also began seeing a therapist. With the help of AA, my sponsor, and my counselor, Art, I began to heal. The more I told Art about how bad I was and how much I had messed up my life, the more he helped me explore my strengths. He taught me that, through it all, I had not only survived; I had also grown as a person and had gained personal strength. I'd learned lessons along the way and helped my children get through it as well. I worked with Art for over two years. I will forever be grateful for my work with this caring and gifted counselor. He inspired me to continue my education.

In the midst of my time working with Art, I completed my internship and became a licensed counselor. I began working as an adolescent counselor for The Right Step, a substance abuse treatment facility in Houston. I loved the work and the people. In 1999, I decided to go into private practice. It was slow in the beginning, but I made enough to support us.

In the summer of 2002, something happened that pushed me to reexamine my spirituality: my sons were in a serious car accident. My older son, Jonathan, was driving; he and his younger brother, Christopher, were going out to lunch for a hamburger. Jonathan had made a left turn when they were broadsided by a pickup truck. They were flown by helicopter to Memorial Hermann Hospital.

The drive to the hospital was surreal. My only thought was that I could not get to them and comfort them. It seemed that everything was moving in slow motion. As I contemplated my children and my total helplessness in the situation, I began to feel God's presence. I prayed fervently that they would be okay. All past issues and struggles paled in comparison to this situation. Nothing else mattered except their well-being.

When I got to the hospital, I went to the emergency room door, and a police officer told me that I could not enter. I looked him square in the eyes and told him that he did not understand; I had two children in there who were badly injured and had just arrived by helicopter, and no one or nothing this side of hell was going to keep me out of there. I told him that he just needed to please step aside. He did.

I heard Jonathan screaming and discovered that he had a broken femur. Medical workers had put weights on his legs as they tried to straighten them out. When I got to him, his main concern was for Christopher. He was afraid that he had killed his beloved little brother. Christopher was across the room. His face was swollen and he had two black eyes. He had a concussion but was awake and alert. He was crying and was worried in turn about his older brother. I was struck by how very caring they were for each other during this trauma.

On Jonathan's armband was the term "Foxtrot." and Christopher's was labeled "Echo." The medical team used these terms because the boys were minors and had not been identified by their parents at the scene of the accident. In my mind, those terms on their armbands magnified how very helpless I felt. I insisted that their names be corrected immediately; it was very important to me that there be no question about their identity. A very thoughtful nurse understood my anxiety over this issue and took care of it right away. The doctors, nurses, and staff at Memorial Hermann Hospital were amazing. I have tremendous respect and gratitude for the emergency team that cared for my children.

Although Christopher's head and face were swollen and he would have some headaches, the brain scans came back normal. and the doctors felt he would be okay. They told me to just keep a close eye on him and give him ibuprofen for the pain and inflammation. The doctors said Jonathan required surgery that would include inserting a rod into his leg.

The next day, after Jonathan came out of surgery and I knew he would be okay, I went to the chapel to be alone. I tried to pray, but the only thing that would come out was "gratitude, gratitude, gratitude." I no longer doubted God; I knew he had been with us through all of it. No longer did I see him as angry or condemning. I understood God to be loving, caring, and compassionate to all people.

When people have been traumatized by religion, it is easy to confuse the love and compassion of God with the fear and dogma of religious teaching. Somehow, people who are stuck in dogma believe that traumatic situations are punishments from God. This situation brought me to the epiphany that there is clearly a distinction between God and religion. I understood that God did not cause this situation, but was certainly there to help us heal and grow from it.

Inspired by this realization, in 2003 I began a master's program at the American Institute of Holistic Theology. This journey was life changing. The curriculum resonated with my soul. I began to see God in a new and bigger way. I loved the study of world religions and metaphysics. These ideas helped me grow tremendously as a person and a counselor. Although compassion had always been one of my strengths, I began seeing that everyone's story has a purpose, and that my job as a counselor is to help my clients in discovering and following that purpose while accepting whatever outcome as being what it is supposed to be.

In 2005, I met Gilbert. When I began telling him about my "stuff" and my imperfections, he stopped me. He told me that I could certainly tell him my story if I wished, but that all he cared about was me and the person I am today. The past did not matter to him. We became good friends. I began to trust him. He never offered me doubt or criticism. He liked my children and they liked him. We married in October 2006.

In 2008, I began my postgraduate work, also through the American Institute of Holistic Theology. I graduated in February 2010 with a PhD in metaphysics. Today, I look in the mirror and love and honor the woman I see there. I am proud of my children and their individual journeys of healing and personal growth.

I owe a debt of gratitude to the many clients who have trusted me, shared their trials, and had the courage to find their way from addiction to peace, power, and a sound mind. Like many of them, I have personally experienced the pain of addiction, as well as the miracle of recovery. I also am grateful for a family who never gave up on me, and for a program that brought me from the darkness and loneliness of addiction to alcohol and toxic relationships, to a life of love, self-respect, and contentment. I wouldn't say that difficulties don't appear from time to time, because that's just life. It just means that recovery has given me the tools to deal with whatever life gives me. With understanding and commitment, healing can and does happen. This book comes from this conviction, from my personal path, and from the experiences of clients.

> With understanding and commitment, healing can and does happen.

In the following chapters, we will delve deeper into the global effects of addiction in people's lives, as well as treatment options and modalities. We will not only look at the traditional medical model of treatment, but also at Twelve Step programs and alternative and complementary methods of coping and healing that have taken a viable place in treatment and recovery.

The stories I share in this book are all true. I have changed some of the names and details in order to protect the anonymity of the people involved. I share them with you because it is vitally important to understand the devastating affects addiction has on people's lives, and to further emphasize the necessity of developing coping skills and tools in order to obtain health and balance. Although it isn't always easy, the lifelong benefits of developing the discipline of a personal plan of recovery combining a sober social support system, such as AA or Narcotics Anonymous (NA), with the empowering holistic methods covered in this book, are immeasurable.

As society moves more toward the idea of wellness, versus simply the treatment of symptoms, we will indeed see a need for the adoption and acceptance of holistic approaches to behavioral, emotional, and physical health and well-being. This was my purpose in writing this book. I wanted to offer an approach that gives people struggling with addictions the tools they need to not only get sober, but to have and maintain wellness in all areas of their lives.

Understanding Addiction

*"We cannot understand anything until we accept it.
Condemnation does not liberate, it oppresses."*
—Carl Jung

During the past fifteen years, working in the field of addictions, I have witnessed many clients enter treatment wanting and expecting to find a way to turn their lives around. Instead, in many cases, they have been given a psychiatric diagnosis and prescribed heavy-duty medications that made them feel worse than when they started.

When we go to a doctor or a hospital for help, we put our trust in those healthcare providers, many times without question. We are not taught as a society to participate in our healthcare or to partner with our physicians in our treatment. Western medicine is primarily based on treatment of the symptoms, not treatment of the underlying problems. It was with this understanding that I created a program that combines the wisdom and structure of the Twelve Steps of Alcoholics Anonymous with self-empowering holistic methods.

By embracing the holistic practices that I cover in this book, I have witnessed numerous clients recover and maintain long-term sobriety, as well as physical, mental, and emotional health. I have seen them accomplish recovery with limited or no use of psychotropic medications. It takes thought and willingness to engage in practices outside of our comfort zones. When making lifestyle changes, such as practicing yoga, developing healthy eating habits, or exploring meditation, we've got to understand that the results are not always immediate. With persistence and consistency, a person can obtain health, and balance in all areas of their life.

Because people with addictions are used to seeking and acquiring immediate gratification, lack of commitment to their own health and wellness and to necessary lifestyle changes is perhaps the number-one reason for their lack of success. It is important to learn that we are all responsible for our own physical, emotional, and mental health. My goal is to teach people different methods of healing and allow them to choose the methods that they most enjoy and find most effective. I have found that when people are involved in their own treatment plans and given options from which to choose, their rates of success increase tremendously.

> Because people with addictions are used to seeking and acquiring immediate gratification, lack of commitment to their own health and wellness and to necessary lifestyle changes is perhaps the number-one reason for their lack of success

Alcoholic Anonymous is one of the most successful methods of arriving at sobriety for people addicted to alcohol and other substances. Perhaps this is true because, in the field of addictions, the modalities of treatment are very limited. AA's success is in large part due to the fellowship and peer support it offers. This is invaluable when people are in the early stages of recovery and have to learn to socialize without the use of substances. Working with an AA sponsor allows people to engage in introspection that is vital for behavioral changes.

Another powerful component of AA is that it provides accountability to another person or group of peers. Peer and social acceptance are significant needs for most people in all stages of their lives. This is the premise on which Dr. Bob Smith and Bill Wilson founded Alcoholics Anonymous many years ago. They found that when alcoholics talk to other alcoholics, they understand one another. They feel accepted, can talk through their problems, and can hold each other accountable.

Although AA has its strong points, it also has its limitations. Some of these limitations include the idea that people must be labeled as addicts or alcoholics for life and must attend meetings on a consistent basis forever in order to remain sober. This limits the idea of personal empowerment and internal strength that holistic methods offer.

Also, the concepts of Alcoholics Anonymous are based on Christianity. For some people, this is certainly a strong point, but for others it is a stumbling block. Although the *Big Book of AA* (AA's guiding text) includes a chapter called "We Agnostics" and attempts to embrace all belief systems, it can be argued that the program's basic structure is fundamentally religious. Steps one through three encourage the idea of powerlessness of the self over alcohol, and the need for redemption by God or a higher power. Steps four and five are based on the Christian ideas of focusing on one's "sins," or character defects, and the concept of confessing one's sins to another human being. The remaining steps include the principles of dying to oneself and being reborn a new person, and the ecclesiastic idea of spreading the "gospel." I'm not saying this religious structure is bad thing; I am just saying that it doesn't work for everyone.

There is a difference between religion and spirituality. Religion is a set of doctrines, rules, and guidelines within which one worships. Spirituality is a relationship with one's higher self or guiding principles. Spirituality can include a deity outside oneself, but it doesn't have to.

Spirituality is a main component of recovery for many people. This is primarily because, through addictions and co-occurring disorders, it is common for people to lose their sense of self and to develop an identity based on shame. In many cases, people's sense of shame is their core issue. This means that they are drinking, taking drugs, or participating in self-destructive behaviors in order to mask the shame that they feel.

Sometimes, shame is a result of religious abuse in people's lives. If someone has participated in and been taught a religion that is fear-based at its core, they often feel resentful and angry towards religion in general.

If this is the case, opening up to the idea of the Twelve Steps may be difficult or even impossible, at least in the beginning. Finding their individual spiritual path is a primary source of healing for such people. Many of the holistic methods covered in this book will lead one to the quiet mind and to one's true and authentic self. This resonates deeply with many people and becomes their spiritual path.

> As society's concepts of spirituality change, treatment must accept and accommodate these ideas. Combining the Western concepts of spirituality espoused in AA's Twelve Steps with the Eastern philosophies of many holistic practices can offer a very well-rounded and balanced approach to treatment, one in which people can express their individuality and choose what empowers them the most.

As society's concepts of spirituality change, treatment must accept and accommodate these ideas. Combining the Western concepts of spirituality espoused in AA's Twelve Steps with the Eastern philosophies of many holistic practices can offer a very well-rounded and balanced approach to treatment, one in which people can express their individuality and choose what empowers them the most.

People enter into recovery seeking peace of mind. While it is true that people cannot recover from the disease of addiction without a willing heart and mind, this is not typically the state in which they enter treatment. Instead, people usually enter treatment because others in their lives are seeking peace of mind because of the chaos and pain created by the addiction. Addicted people enter treatment because they have been given an ultimatum by their loved ones, by the court, or by their employers.

Sometimes, people do come to treatment because they are tired of all the physical, emotional, legal, financial, mental, and social consequences of their addictions. In other words, they are sick and tired of being sick and tired.

For our purposes, alcoholism and addiction are the same thing; the words are interchangeable. Addiction to alcohol, drugs, and even certain behaviors, such as anger, criminal behavior, sex, and food, occurs in the brain. Addiction of any kind is driven by the release of endorphins in the brain brought on by the drug or behavior and the compulsive need to repeat the behavior in order to feel comfortable or normal. However, as addiction progresses, the end result becomes more and more uncomfortable and even painful.

From the addicts' perspectives, they are using the objects of their addictions to feel better, and all behavior is about feeling better. It seems that the more their lives begin to fall apart because of the addiction, the more tightly the addiction grips them. Because the addiction is their primary way of coping with life, they are terrified of living without it. A recovery process that involves both the Twelve Steps and self-empowering holistic methods teaches people to unlearn self-destructive thoughts and behaviors and relearn new, more effective ways of living.

Definition

Let's begin with a basic understanding of addiction. Addiction can be defined as a pathological, love and trust relationship with a chemical, person, object, or behavior. The behavior is pathological because it is obsessive, compulsive, and maladaptive in nature. In other words, it isn't good for you, and it creates chaos in your life. It is characterized in terms of love and trust because addicts know that when they drink, take the drug, or

> Addiction can be defined as a pathological, love and trust relationship with a chemical, person, object, or behavior.

participate in the behavior, they will have an immediate, positive payoff or sense of relief.

Addiction is a relationship because it becomes part of every facet of people's lives: who they choose to be friends with, where they go, how they celebrate, how they relax, how they cope with stress, and so forth. When we look at this definition, we can see that one can be addicted to many things besides alcohol or drugs. One can be addicted to anger, food, sex, certain people, gambling, or shopping. People can even be addicted to the addiction itself; in other words, sometimes people are addicted to the sense of powerlessness that identifying themselves as "addicts" creates. Often, loved ones in the addicts' lives become so vested into trying to control or stop the addiction that they become addicted to the drama and insanity the addiction creates. When life becomes balanced, or "normal," this becomes strange and uncomfortable, even boring.

When people have an addiction, they are unable to resist the compulsion to take the drug, drink the alcohol, or participate in the behavior, even when anticipating negative consequences. They will experience physical or psychological withdrawal symptoms if abruptly deprived of the chemical or the behavior. For instance, people who are addicted to anger will feel very uncomfortable when learning to accept irritations without angry or controlling behaviors. Sometimes people will experience stomach pains, shortness of breath, or the sensation of tightness across the temples when learning to respond in a manner that is new and inconsistent with their habitual nature. Remember, all behavior is about feeling better, so acting contradictory to what feels better is very difficult.

When people are withdrawing from drugs or alcohol, they often feel nauseated, irritable, and discontent. Their natural coping method is to drink or use drugs, and they know that if they do, they will immediately feel better, even if the feeling is temporary and will be followed by negative consequences. The urge to use to feel better is so powerful that the behavior becomes compulsive. An understanding of addiction, a desire to change the behavior, and a strong support system are all vital to people in treatment and recovery.

Addiction, whether chemical or behavioral, works on a continuum. Since addiction is progressive in nature, even the mildest forms of addiction can, without intervention, lead to serious dependence, illness, or perhaps even death.

Stages

Addiction to chemicals begins with the primary stage of occasional, recreational use. Not everyone who uses alcohol or drugs is dependent on them. Some people become dependent on substances more quickly and easily than other people. That said, anyone who uses mind-altering, mood-altering substances for long enough and in enough quantity will develop a tolerance and will become dependent on them. Stemming from different causes, addiction to behaviors will also follow a continuum and create chaos and pain in one's life.

The next stage of the continuum of addiction is the progressive stage. In this stage, people become more preoccupied with how to obtain the drug and how they will feel when they use it. Most social functions become centered around drinking or drug use. Friendships and peer groups begin to change. Family members and friends begin to see behavioral changes. These changes may include sleeping more or less, poor appetite and eating habits, and lack of attention to hygiene and personal appearance. Mood swings may also become more pronounced.

The progressive stage of addiction is characterized by obsession and compulsion. People may try to change their drinking or using patterns. They may tell themselves, "I'll only have a couple of drinks," only to find that once they start drinking or using they cannot quit until they become intoxicated and embarrass themselves or pass out. During this stage of addiction, defense mechanisms become prevalent. People may begin to downplay or hide their drinking. Defensive behaviors become more common as friends and family become concerned and question the changes that they see.

Addicted people begin to experience blackouts, instances in which they wake up the next day not remembering what they said or did the night before. Blackouts often occur without intervals of unconsciousness. People are awake, talking, and behaving without being aware of what they are doing. The next day, they may have little or no memory of the experience. This creates embarrassment and, often, a deep sense of shame. Blackouts are signs that addiction is developing or progressing.

Addictions now begin to take on lives of their own. Peoples' lifestyles begin to break down. As the addicted lifestyle becomes more comfortable or ordinary to them, they are more likely to enter compromising situations. People may have encounters with the law, perhaps in the form of DWIs, public intoxication, or possession charges. Relationships begin to be taxed as addicted people begin to lie about drug or alcohol use. As the addiction progresses, people begin to lose more and more in their lives.

The next phase of the addiction is called the chronic stage. At this point, people are at a crossroads in their lives. What makes this stage so difficult is that the addiction is now in control. Addicted people have lost identification with their true selves; they now identify with their addiction. It is their world. They sometimes feel that if they use again they will die, and if they don't, they will die. They become trapped in endless cycles of denial, pain, and above all, shame. To deal with the shame, they begin the cycle of denial and use again. This cycle will repeat itself over and over again unless there is an intervention of some sort. Without intervention, either by the addict themselves or by someone else, the chronic stage of addiction will end in jail, or possibly even death.

Causes

The causes of addiction are difficult for most people to understand. Addiction is insidious because one of its chief characteristics is denial. Denial is different than lying. When people lie, they know they are lying. When people are in denial, they don't realize it. It seems that everyone around addicted people can clearly see what the addicts themselves cannot see. No one sets out to become addicted, and no one wants to be an addict. No one woke up one morning and said, "I think I want to be a drug addict," or, "I think I'd like to be an alcoholic." In fact, when people hear the terms "drug addict" or "alcoholic" in reference to themselves, they typically become offended and perhaps defensive, even if deep down they know there is a problem.

Addiction does not begin because people are depressed, running away from something, or have had bad parenting. True, these issues may be part of people's lives and may have occurred along the way for various reasons. These issues may even be contributing factors to addiction. But the true cause of addiction lies in how the brain reacts to substances; addiction happens in the brain.

When some people use mind-altering substances, they feel a little intoxicated and stop; they have a red light in their brains, if you will. In contrast, people who have a tendency toward addiction react differently. When alcohol or drugs enter their systems, their brains are flooded with endorphins. Such people have this reaction, if not the first time they use, then very early in the primary stage of addiction. They have no red stoplight, only a green light. To such people, being high or being drunk feels normal. When people recall the beginning stages of their use, they will have very fond memories of the sensation of intoxication. Even when they are in emotional or physical pain as a result of their addiction, they will still chase the feeling of intoxication. It is as if they are on a rollercoaster and can't get off. When alcoholics drink or use drugs, a craving begins and does not allow them to moderate their use.

An addiction can, and often does, begin with the use of prescription medications. These medications are typically given for pain or anxiety management, and fall into the categories of opiates and benzodiazepines. People can develop a tolerance to these drugs quickly. Tolerance simply means that it takes more of the drug to achieve the same effect. So, in order to manage the pain or anxiety, people need to take more and more of the drug. When they try to get off the drug, they tend to be quite physically sick and have joint and muscle aches, sometimes accompanied by nausea and diarrhea. This in turn signals the brain to take more of the drug to alleviate the symptoms. Not only does the brain know the drug will relieve the pain; it also recalls the euphoric effect of the drug. The positive payoff is cemented in the brain, and the addiction to the drug develops strength.

Demographics

Addiction crosses all socioeconomic, racial and religious boundaries. For example, just because a person comes from a financially privileged background doesn't mean they are less vulnerable to addiction.

At one time, it was believed that women were less susceptible to addiction than men. Research has shown that this is not true. I will not give percentages here, because I feel they are inaccurate and change all the time because of different methods of measurement and social contributing factors. Nonetheless, it is safe to say that the percentage of women seeking treatment for substance abuse has risen dramatically over the past few years.

Another evident societal change is that the onset age of substance abuse has lowered dramatically over the years. When I began working in the field of addiction fifteen years ago, the common age of onset reported in psychosocial assessments was thirteen or fourteen. Today, I see the onset of addiction in clients as young as nine or ten years old. Many social factors point to this issue. Today, the divorce and blended family rates are much higher than they were even twenty years ago. There are many single-parent households in which children are not adequately supervised. Many times, these parents become focused on their new and developing social lives and lose sight of what is happening with their children and the influences being brought into their homes.

I should also note that the rate of addiction to pain medication (opiates) in particular has rapidly risen in recent years. One contributing factor has been the increasing ease of access to narcotics, especially through so-called pain clinics, which are found in great numbers in many cities and towns. In many cases, the doctors in these clinics work on a cash-only basis and are partnered with a "pharmacy" that the patient is required to use. Many clients have told me that obtaining prescriptions for large quantities of very powerful narcotics was quite simple at these clinics. All that is necessary is to say, "I have headaches," or "My back hurts." When patients ask to use something less powerful, many are discouraged from doing so. Thankfully, the drug enforcement agencies have been cracking down on these facilities, and regulations are becoming stricter. Many times these types of clinics do not stay in business for very long. They will settle in a place, make a large amount of money, and close up shop before they get into trouble.

Many people have also told me that they became addicted to narcotics by obtaining them from the Internet. All that was required was for them to fill out a form online. Then, a doctor, whom they had never seen in person, approved the prescription based on the symptoms described, and the medication was delivered to their doorstep via courier.

JOHN

John was a successful businessman who came to me seeking treatment because he was struggling with an addiction to hydrocodone. He owned and operated an accounting and bookkeeping firm. His wife accompanied him to the original assessment. John reported that he was using between fifty and sixty pills daily and had been doing so for the past year and a half. He explained that he had started using them to treat a golf-related back injury. He said that he truly wanted to get off of the narcotics, but they gave him the energy to accomplish the tasks he wanted to get done, and he was very afraid of the withdrawal symptoms that he had experienced when trying to get off of them by himself. John's wife reported that he had become secretive and was no longer affectionate. She also explained that she was angry and concerned because he had spent vast amounts of money paying for his addiction. John was encouraged to go into inpatient and residential treatment, where he could detox safely under the supervision of a medical team and remove himself from an environment in which it was so easy for him to obtain the drugs. My concern was that, while in active or even post-acute withdrawal, the temptation to buy a prescription would be too great. He needed help.

Unfortunately, John refused these options, and instead chose to take medication to help alleviate the withdrawal symptoms without complementary treatment. What he did not do was develop the coping skills necessary to deal with the stressors of work, the marital problems incurred by his addiction, and the behavioral patterns he had developed in order to maintain his addiction. As both time and his addiction progressed, John began stealing money from his clients and his company's investors. He is now divorced from his wife, his company is bankrupt, and he is serving ten years in federal prison because of the illegal behaviors he developed in order to feed his addiction. I have received several letters from John telling me how much he regrets not going into treatment and how sad he is about losing his wife and hurting so many people. When John leaves prison, he will be close to sixty years old with nothing to his name and will no longer be allowed to work in his chosen profession. He will have to learn new means of supporting himself and a new way of living.

We may be tempted to stand in judgment of John; after all, his decisions hurt many people. Addiction drives many people to make decisions that are outside their principles and their basic beliefs of right and wrong. When one is addicted to a drug, the compulsion to obtain and use the drug often overpowers one's sense of integrity. I am not saying addiction is an excuse for bad behavior; there are consequences in life for all of our decisions, both good and bad. I am saying that addiction, left untreated, very often leads to heartbreaking results. My motivation for this book is to offer genuine hope for the struggling addict and the tools for life-long recovery and peace of mind.

Withdrawal Treatment

Thankfully, research has given us options for helping people get off of highly addictive pain medications without the painful withdrawal symptoms. Although I advocate that clients take the least amount of any drug possible to reach the highest good, there is a time and place for medications. Withdrawal from opiates in particular can be so painful and uncomfortable that it is very difficult to get past the detoxification stage of recovery. However, it must be stressed that many medications used for detoxification comfort can be addictive and must be monitored closely by a physician who is trained specifically to use them. It is equally important that these medications are used in conjunction with psychological and complementary approaches for long-term recovery.

A common drug used by addictionologists and other physicians for opiate withdrawal is buprenorphine, sold under the trade name Suboxone. Buprenorphine works by binding to the same receptors in the brain as the opioid drug. It mimics the effects of other opiates by alleviating cravings and withdrawal symptoms. Most patients feel better within an hour of taking buprenorphine.

Although withdrawal from opiates can be very uncomfortable and will often result in relapse if there isn't help with the discomfort, withdrawal isn't life-threatening. Deaths associated with opiate addiction occur because of overdoses; doses taken in combination with alcohol or benzodiazepines can cause respiratory shutdown, life-style consequences such as septicemia (blood infections), HIV, and hepatitis C, or accidents. The problem with buprenorphine and other drugs used to treat withdrawal symptoms is that, if not monitored closely, they can become addictive as well. Withdrawal from them can be a harsh process.

This book offers alternatives that can help with withdrawal and post-acute withdrawal for those who choose not to take medication. In particular, deep, conscious breathing, body scans, and guided imagery are quite effective in easing the pain and discomfort of withdrawal. The results of such practices in our program have been outstanding.

We must also look at the alarming rate at which people are prescribed anti-anxiety, antidepressant, antipsychotic, and pain medications, not to mention the stimulant drugs given for attention deficit disorder and weight management. This is not to say that such medications are never appropriate, but rather that, as healthcare providers, we over-diagnose and over-prescribe these medications. We tend to focus on alleviating the symptoms instead of the problems. In doing so, we have created a generation—or two—of addicts. We have not taught people to cope with the stressors of life, but rather to escape from them.

Withdrawal from alcohol or benzodiazepines, on the other hand, can be very dangerous and can cause seizures, delirium tremors, hallucinations, and even death. When withdrawing from either of these substances, physicians who are familiar with addiction should monitor people. Many healthcare professionals are only minimally trained in the area of addiction, so people struggling with addictions should make sure that their healthcare providers have an adequate understanding of addiction and the detoxification and withdrawal process.

As a matter of responsible practice, when people are withdrawing from benzodiazepines or large quantities of alcohol, I require them to detoxify under the care of a medical doctor. When they are safely detoxified and past the danger of seizures or death, I begin working with them on what is referred to as post-acute withdrawal. During this period of time, people experience such symptoms such as anxiousness, nervousness, and even some physical pain. In addition to deep breathing, we use meditation, yoga, guided imagery, and brainwave synchronization to address these symptoms, with very good results.

Holistic practices are not only valuable during acute and post-acute withdrawal; they also empower people with tools for ongoing sobriety and personal wellness.

Beyond Withdrawal

Treatment is usually necessary to help people lessen their affinities for intoxication. Because all behaviors are about feeling better, they must learn new, effective ways of having fun and feeling peaceful. Beyond physically managing withdrawal, people must learn coping skills and alternative methods for pain and anxiety management. Addicts have to learn to live in a whole new way. They have to learn to relax, celebrate, and enjoy life without the use of substances, even when those around them use. This is true no matter what mind-altering, mood-altering substances people are addicted to.

Here, it must be stressed that healing and recovery *can* happen. The field of addiction studies and treatment has come a long way in understanding the multifaceted effects of this devastating disease, especially from a psychosocial perspective. I personally see miracles happen all the time when people do the work of recovery and find mental, emotional, physical, and spiritual health.

2

Addiction: A Family Affair

"Forgiveness is a rebirth of hope, a reorganization of thought, and a reconstruction of dreams. Once forgiving begins, dreams can be rebuilt. When forgiving is complete, meaning has been extracted from the worst of experiences and used to create a new set of moral rules and a new interpretation of life events."
—Beverly Flanigan

*L*et us now take our understanding of addiction to the next level. Addiction not only affects people with the addiction; it also affects everyone they are in relationships with. Often those closest to addicted people become addicted to the addiction. Their thoughts and behaviors become obsessive and compulsive as well. They are in a constant state of turmoil, never knowing what to expect. Loved ones are always thinking about the addiction and will become hyper-vigilant in trying to stop or control the addict's behaviors and their resulting consequences.

Sometimes, spouses, parents, or children have such a fear of abandonment that they become enabling, making excuses and developing behaviors that keep a semblance of peace in the family. If this continues, loved ones will begin to lose their sense of selves. Families' lives begin to revolve around addicts and their addictions. I call this "doing the dance": the addicts do one thing, and the partners or families react in a certain way to counteract the effects. Over time, this behavior becomes a pattern, one that is difficult to recognize or change.

> Addiction not only affects people with the addiction; it also affects everyone they are in relationships with. Often those closest to addicted people become addicted to the addiction.

People who are not alcoholics think, *"Why don't they just stop? I can,"* or, *"If our relationship were important to her, she would quit,"* or, *"If he loved the kids, he wouldn't use drugs."* It seems insane that a person would lose so much, endure so much chaos and pain, and *still* continue to use—and indeed, it is insane. It is often said that until a person hits the bottom they will not change. The loved ones say, "My God, how far down is the bottom?"

I have been an addictions counselor for many years. I love my work and can't imagine another calling. That said, I think it's important to acknowledge that, although there are many stories that have positive outcomes, there are also those that end in heartbreak. Some end with jail, and some end with death.

AARON

Aaron was a twenty-year-old man in treatment at our clinic for addiction to multiple substances. Aaron was vibrant, handsome, and extremely talented. He was a musician and a writer and was quite popular with his peer group. He was the only child of Diane and Jay.

Aaron grew up enjoying the good things in life. He openly talked about how much he loved his mom and her cooking. He chatted about the fun times he enjoyed with his dad, fishing and riding dirt bikes.

At the time of his admission to treatment, Aaron related that his relationship with his parents had become strained. He reported that he had been using marijuana regularly for the past five years. In addition, he had been using alcohol regularly for the past two years. Six months prior to admittance to treatment, Aaron's drug use had escalated to the abuse of benzodiazepines and muscle relaxers. Although he had been hospitalized for a drug overdose, he was in denial about the seriousness of his addiction. His parents were extremely worried, and Aaron reported that he and his parents had had numerous arguments about his drug use.

Aaron agreed to treatment and said he really wanted to improve his relationship with his parents. He was consistent in attendance and participated well in group therapy. His parents attended family group regularly. Aaron was a musician and loved to play the blues and rock and roll. He identified strongly with Jimi Hendrix and Stevie Ray Vaughan, and he loved to play their music. Both artists were drug addicts. Jimi Hendrix died of a drug overdose. Aaron vowed that he would not follow that example. During several family sessions, Aaron agreed to be sober and refrain from all drug and alcohol use. He mentioned that when he was sober, he felt better and was more productive. His parents reported that Aaron was happier and that their communication as a family had improved greatly.

However, during treatment, Aaron found it difficult to refrain from marijuana use. From his perspective, it was no big deal. After Aaron completed treatment, his parents continued to come to family group for ongoing support. Aaron continued to attend group meetings sporadically.

At the time of this writing, Aaron's parents are planning his memorial service. He had renewed his acquaintances with his drug-using friends, and one Saturday he bought some Xanax and hydrocodone. After having an enjoyable dinner with his mother, he decided to get high and go out and party with his friends. Two blocks from home, he lost control of his car and hit a light pole. He died instantly.

ALLISON

Allison was a thirty-six-year-old woman who entered treatment because she had developed an addiction to prescription pain medication, which she received for migraine headaches. Allison had struggled with migraines for much of her life, and they escalated in frequency and intensity when she became pregnant with her son, Jimmy. Allison also related that she had struggled with severe postpartum depression, which was treated with antidepressants.

Prior to her son's birth, Allison worked as a paramedic and loved helping people. This was evident in the compassion she displayed to her group peers while in treatment. Allison had a beautiful, vibrant spirit. She was a ballerina and loved to dance. In addition, she loved her husband, Sam, with a passion. She enjoyed her large extended family and talked about them endlessly.

Although there were trips to the emergency room for pain management throughout her adult life, the emergency room visits became more frequent as her dependency on pain medication increased. When Allison would try to get off of the pain medication, she would experience muscle aches and nausea. This would increase her anxiety and stress, and would often trigger a headache. As time progressed, so did the cycle of addiction.

Allison's husband, Sam, attended Al-Anon meetings on a regular basis. He tried to set appropriate boundaries with Allison while also being sympathetic to her pain. Allison attended an outpatient program and Twelve Step meetings, but after time, she began to make excuses for missing meetings.

As her addiction progressed, Allison discovered the use of inhalants. She began huffing canned air in order to achieve a euphoric effect. She was then admitted to a psychiatric residential treatment program, where she was treated for her addiction as well as her depression. She stayed for forty five days. During treatment, Allison learned coping skills and began to understand the seriousness of her addiction.

While in treatment, and for a period of time afterward, Allison's headaches became less frequent and less severe. She attended Twelve Step meetings and an aftercare group. Her relationships became healthier and more balanced. She related that she was happy and felt a newfound sense of hope and freedom.

After a short period of time, however, Allison stopped going to meetings and began isolating herself. She then began buying and huffing canned air again. Her headaches increased, as did her use of opiates. The cycle began again, only this time with greater intensity. When her son was six years old, two weeks before Christmas, Allison was found dead in a hotel room. She had overdosed on canned air and pain medication. Her family was devastated. I will always remember watching her husband and little boy closing the door on the hearse as they prepared to take her to the cemetery. The sadness of that moment will be etched in their hearts and in my mind forever.

Addiction is a painful and deadly disease that affects the brain, the heart, and the soul of a person. It affects individuals, families, and societies. It has no boundaries. As a counselor, I have seen numerous people die from this disease. I have seen people go to jail again and again, always vowing to break the cycle. Clients have looked me in the eyes and begged me not to give up on them, and I never do give up. I have watched parents, grandparents, spouses, and children cry and helplessly wring their hands as they watch the ones they love spiral into the insanity of addiction. Honestly, I have done the same. But what keep me going are the miracles. Healing does happen. With commitment to a program of recovery, and with support, people with addictions can live a productive and happy life.

Because of the component of denial, recovery is more difficult for some people than others. Recovery requires honesty, open-mindedness, and a willingness to change—not only on the part of addicts, but on the part of loved ones as well. Many times, parents or loved ones feel that they have done something wrong, or that there must be a deep underlying issue that has caused the addiction. Although it is true that emotionally healthy people do not participate in self-destructive behavior, addiction happens because the positive payoff in the brain induced by the substance overpowers the

> Recovery requires honesty, open-mindedness, and a willingness to change—not only on the part of addicts, but on the part of loved ones as well.

negative consequences of the use. For some people, this process will continue until the negative consequences outweigh the positive payoffs.

False Beliefs

Our mind has a way of remembering the good things and suppressing things that are too painful or embarrassing to face.

When alcoholics consider giving up alcohol, they typically experience an internal power struggle between the reality of the situation and their own false beliefs or denials. The addicted mind says, *"If I stop drinking, I won't have fun anymore."*

The sober mind says, *"This alcohol is not good for you. It will hurt you and eventually kill you."*

And then the addicted mind says, *"Yes, I know, but I'll miss going to the club."* It goes on to say such things as:

- *"I can control it. I'll drink less."*
- *"I won't drink strong liquor; I'll just drink beer."*
- *"How can I eat Italian food without a good merlot?"*
- *"What about those wonderful nights of drinking and dancing and making love?"*
- *"What if I'm not as much fun to my husband? Will he leave me?"*
- *"I make a great brisket. How can I do that without beer?"*

The mind has a way of remembering when the alcohol *did* work, and forgetting about, or minimizing, all the times when it didn't. The brain remembers the relaxation and euphoria of the marijuana or the opiates. It remembers getting high with friends, listening to good music, and having fun. The mind remembers smoking and feeling the day's stress slip away.

The addicted mind doesn't see what other people see. The addicted mind doesn't say, *"I've quit school or failed because I can't focus or concentrate and would rather just get high."* The addicted mind says, *"School is dumb anyway and the teacher was an idiot."* The addicted mind doesn't say, *"I've lost my job and can't pay my bills because I smoked pot, took those pills, and maybe created a liability at work that my employer shouldn't tolerate."* Instead, the addicted brain will say, *"That boss was unfair. He should've minded his own business. I was treated badly, so forget them. I'm better off without that job."*

If the person gets arrested for possession of illegal substances, the addicted mind will not say, *"I broke the law, I should pay this consequence."* The addicted mind will say, *"That cop or judge has no right to run my life and tell me what I can or cannot do. Anyway, I was stopped and searched unfairly. I wasn't that high or drunk anyway. My attorney will get the tape and prove it."*

Many times, as the addiction progresses, families will spend vast amounts of money bailing addicts out. To rationalize these actions, families will think things like, *"After all, if she has a record, her life is ruined."* They also think to themselves, *"If he loved and respected me, he would see what we have paid and how hard this is for us."*

However, when addicts face no consequences, the addiction is cemented further. When other people have picked up the pieces, addicts have no reason to see the extent of their problems. Denial keeps the addict from seeing the whole picture. It is not until they have to take responsibility for the consequences of their behaviors; including financial, legal, emotional, and physical problems, that there is an incentive to change.

> Denial keeps the addict from seeing the whole picture. It is not until they have to take responsibility for the consequences of their behaviors; including financial, legal, emotional, and physical problems, that there is an incentive to change.

Obviously, as the addict's lifestyle begin to break down, there is more stress in their lives. Now, they are drinking or using drugs to deal with the stress. When relationships become fractured, when finances become strained, when legal issues occur, and when embarrassing situations crop up, self-esteem plummets.

It would seem that, at this point, a person would want to change. But it isn't that simple. As our self-esteem lowers, our addicted minds create false belief systems to protect us, including:

- *"It isn't hurting anyone."*
- *"I'm in control of this."*
- *"No one has a right to tell me what to do."*
- *"I'm sexy when I drink."*

- *"I'm tough."*
- *"I'm a sweet drunk."*
- *"I have a right to be angry!"*
- *"I'm cool."*
- *"I'm a smart businessman."*
- *"I'm a great husband, father, wife, or mother."*
- *"I'm just kicking back!"*

The addict begins to manipulate others to believe what they want so desperately to believe. Sometimes these false beliefs develop into personality disorders like narcissism, borderline personality disorders, and antisocial personality disorders.

As addictions progress, the chaos and pain increases, as do the defense mechanisms. Although well-meaning, family members and friends just make the problems worse when they shield the addict from the consequences of their addictions.

As the chaos increases, the addiction takes on a life of its own. Family members become worried and afraid of losing their loved one. They will adopt behaviors in order to cope with the insanity around them. Just as addicts have strong systems of denial, so do family members. Parents, spouses, and children will make excuses for addicts. Family members learn to walk on eggshells to keep the peace and to keep addicts from acting out, often becoming so focused on the addiction that they develop what is referred to as codependency.

Codependency

Codependency is sometimes confused with dependency on another person. In reality, it is the opposite. It means meeting the other person's needs to the exclusion of your own. Codependent people are so vested in keeping the peace and creating a sense of stability that they will forego their own needs. Many times, they will reach a point at which they no longer know who they are or what they want in life. Sometimes this behavior affects multiple generations in families. When people enter treatment

> Codependency is sometimes confused with dependency on another person. In reality, it is the opposite. It means meeting the other person's needs to the exclusion of your own

for addiction, it is imperative for their families to participate in order to learn new boundaries and coping skills for themselves.

Codependents are not always honest about what they see, hear, and feel. They see their relationships based on what they want them to be, instead of reality. For example, parents may have plenty of evidence that their sons or daughters are using drugs and behaving in dangerous or dishonest manners. In some cases, the parents are so afraid of their children's anger or rejection—or so afraid of feeling like failed parents—that they will see their children as "just having fun" or "just being normal teenagers." Instead of taking on parenting roles, parents may try to be their children's best friends and allow certain behaviors that are inappropriate or even illegal. But just because certain behaviors, such as illegal drug use or disrespectful language, are common, that does not make them "normal" or appropriate.

Teenagers do not need their parents to be their best friends. They need them to be parents. It is not just the job of a parent to raise children, but to raise young adults who have the tools and self-esteem to be able to function well in society. This means they need to be taught healthy boundaries and learn the difference between acceptable and unacceptable behaviors. When parents model inappropriate or illegal behavior, they can expect their children to follow their examples. If parents do not have good personal boundaries, it will be much more difficult for their children to learn good boundaries for themselves and in their relationships with other people.

> It is not just the job of a parent to raise children, but to raise young adults who have the tools and self-esteem to be able to function well in society.

In many cases, people who are codependent come from alcoholic or addicted families. They've learned to live by certain rules that stem from defense mechanisms they used as children to cope with the uncertainties and chaos in the family system, rules like:

- *Don't rock the boat.*
- *Lie low or you might get hurt.*
- *Don't have feelings.*
- *Keep the family secret.*
- *Don't trust others.*

We carry our childhood experiences into our adult lives, including the coping and defense mechanisms that we've developed. These have been our "normal." We may say and believe that we will live differently, but childhood patterns are very difficult to break. The family we grew up in is where we developed our sense of belonging and our sense of self. The more dysfunctional the family, the more difficult it is for children to develop healthy, functional relationships throughout their lives.

One of the most difficult issues in treatment is distinguishing between enabling and supportive behavior. The distinguishing factor between the two is that enabling behavior rationalizes, minimizes, or denies the seriousness of the addiction. Enabling is when loved ones allow or contribute to behaviors that keep the addiction progressing. Enabling is making excuses for someone who is acting irresponsibly. Enablers take on responsibilities that addicted people are able to do for themselves and help with the tasks of daily life—work, financial obligations, and so forth.

In contrast, supportive behavior encourages people to reach their highest potential; to become creative and self-sufficient. People in recovery need their families and loved ones to be compassionate and supportive of their recovery efforts. They will need time to go to Twelve Step meetings, develop spiritual practices, and focus on their physical and emotional health. Being supportive of a person in recovery is not always easy because of the time it takes away from family and friends, especially in the beginning. But, in time, the benefits of being supportive far outweigh the inconveniences.

One of the most difficult tasks of recovery, whether we are addicts or codependents, is to face our issues from childhood and how they affect our lives today. Part of this difficulty is due to a sense of loyalty to our families; we fear betraying them if we look at the negative aspects of our childhoods openly and honestly. I have found it most beneficial to help people understand that it isn't about betrayal or being disloyal; that, in fact, our parents did the best they could with where they were at the time. The truth is, though, that it is our responsibility to define our lives and lead them to the best of our abilities. We have the power to break old, dysfunctional patterns of behavior if we can be honest, open-minded, and forgiving.

We cannot change the past, but we can change our view of it. We can choose to be angry, bitter, and resentful, or we can choose to turn our pasts into learning experiences. We can take with us what worked well, and we can let go of what did not. In other words, we can eat the meat and spit out the bones.

It can be a very healing process to see our parents and grandparents from a compassionate perspective; to understand that they, too, were products of their pasts and that they experienced their own wounds. Coming from a place of compassion is healing, not only for those who came before us, but for ourselves and for future generations. As we heal, we develop healthy boundaries and coping methods. When we base our lives on love, compassion, self-respect, and respect toward others, we will indeed model those behaviors for our children and for those around us.

> Coming from a place of compassion is healing, not only for those who came before us, but for ourselves and for future generations.

3

Toxic Relationships

"True Love is not a painful obsession. It is not taking a hostage or being a hostage. It is not all-consuming, isolating, or constricting. Unfortunately the type of love most of us learned about as children is in fact an addiction, a form of toxic love."
—Robert Burney

*M*any people who struggle with addictions are spiritually and emotionally bankrupt. They do not love themselves, and typically believe that they have made so many mistakes that even God cannot love them. It is common for people with chemical addictions to have histories of toxic relationships, and for them to be perplexed about why they get hurt again and again, and why they hurt others again and again.

When we do not feel lovable, it is impossible to accept love or to give love in a healthy way. People who struggle with addictions do not feel lovable, but want and need love desperately. This is a core issue for many people, and if it is not addressed in the treatment and recovery process, it is very likely to lead to more hurt and pain and to increase the risk of relapse. Twelve Step programs offer sober social support groups, but not treatment. Most AA groups recommend that people early in recovery avoid getting into relationships of any kind in the first year of sobriety, and it is highly frowned upon for people in Twelve Step meetings to date each other.

Although sponsorship is a very important part of a Twelve Step support group and offers much needed assistance and support to the recovering person, it is appropriate that Twelve Step programs do not address underlying psychological issues, because Twelve Step sponsors are not therapists. Most sponsors have not been taught to deal with the underlying, core issues that drive some of the problems that co-occur with addictions. I would go so far as to say that it would be irresponsible and sometimes dangerous for them to try. For example, sometimes addicts or alcoholics have attachment disorders, and they may develop strong and even unhealthy attachments to their sponsors. Perhaps they are bipolar or have borderline personality disorder, both of which are common among addicted people. If not treated appropriately, the outcomes of such disorders can be disastrous.

Given the limitations of AA, what I propose is a complementary approach that includes:

- The sober social support and accountability that AA offers.
- The holistic approaches that I offer in this book.
- Solution-focused talk therapy.
- Group counseling.
- Multi-family group counseling.

The more vested people are in addictions of any kind, the more distanced they become from their true and authentic self. It is as if they have a gaping hole in the middle of their soul. The more they drink, use drugs, have sex, spend money, or engage in whatever behavior they use to cope, the more unsatisfied they become. This is particularly true when chemical

> The more vested people are in addictions of any kind, the more distanced they become from their true and authentic self.

addictions are coupled with attachment disorders. The more unsatisfied people feel, the more they grasp for the acceptance of others. The words "I love you" come to mean "I need you," and progress to "I own you." People may be very sincere when they say, "I love you," but their love is typically self-serving and about making themselves feel accepted. It is said that water seeks its level. The more toxic addicted people become, the more toxic their relationships become. This is true for all relationships, not just sexual and romantic ones, An important part of the recovery process is learning what healthy relationships consist of. Healthy relationships are based on trust, honesty, and appropriate boundaries.

Fear of Rejection

An unhealthy relationship does not understand intimacy and is typically based on a deep fear of abandonment or rejection at its core. In many cases, this is evident in one extreme or the other. On one end of the spectrum, people will keep others at arm's length and will not be able to show their true feelings. Their inner belief system says, *"If I let you get too close, you might see who I really am…and you might not like what you see."* Since we project onto others what we believe about ourselves, it's frightening for people with poor self-image to allow others to see their true selves. Although people with poor self-image may want desperately to be close to others, their strong fear of abandonment does not allow such vulnerability. Those who love them, including spouses and children, often feel that they are on the outside, knocking and trying to get in, but no one will answer the door.

Sometimes fear of abandonment and rejection shows itself in a different way. People who fear abandonment sometimes become emotionally and mentally abusive, although they may not see it that way. They have a constant need for affirmation and attention, to the point that they become suffocating to their loved ones. At this point, the people they are in relationships with become the objects of an addiction to them. Their relationships will take on an obsessive and controlling nature; they will believe their partners are responsible for their emotional well-being, and will do and say everything they can to make sure the other person meets their needs. Addicts will always be fearful, wondering where their spouses are, who they are talking to, what they are saying, or what they are doing. They become bulldozers in their relationships.

People addicted to toxic relationships are so sure that they will be left or mistreated that they create the scenario in their mind, and will look for clues to confirm their worst fears. The relationship moves from states of idealization to devaluation, and those in relationships with them will never know where they stand.

> People addicted to toxic relationships are so sure that they will be left or mistreated that they create the scenario in their mind, and will look for clues to confirm their worst fears.

Just as chemical addictions are progressive in nature, so, too, are toxic relationships. I have used the terms "addict" and "partner" to ease the discussion, but in actuality, both people in an abusive, toxic relationship become addicted to the drama and intensity. A more appropriate term than "partner" would be "codependent." Codependents take on the emotional—and often the physical and financial—responsibilities in the relationship. In other words, codependents become doormats in relationships. It is interesting that bulldozers attract doormats, and doormats attract bulldozers. Neither have a healthy sense of self or an understanding of a mature, responsible relationship. They will each attract people into their lives who meet their current belief system of what a relationship "should" be.

When codependents try to communicate or stand up for themselves, their partners will become emotionally, mentally, or even physically aggressive. They will sometimes resort to childlike behaviors, such as name-calling, sarcasm, or pouting. Sometimes, both partners take on similar, immature behaviors. Each will genuinely believe that he or she is right, and will tell the other person that they are crazy or mentally ill if they disagree with him or her. Both people will believe that they, themselves, are in fact the victim.

In an increasingly toxic relationship, if one person tries to leave or end the relationship, the other person will say things like, "If you leave me, I'll have no reason to get sober or change." They may even threaten to kill themselves. Because their partners have little or no self-esteem (if they did, they wouldn't be in such a relationship), they will feel a sense of obligation to stay. Each time either partner tries to leave, the violence tends to increase. This obsession and need to control becomes so powerful that the addict, or codependent, or both, will try to control everyone around them. They will blame everyone else for their own miseries.

As you can see, in actuality, both partners become addicted to the intensity and drama of their toxic relationships. The codependent becomes more enmeshed, believing that it is their responsibility to keep the addict happy, or at least keep them from harming themselves or others. This belief feeds the codependent's need to be needed and falsely boosts their self-esteem. It is necessary to understand that healthy people are not in relationships with toxic people. If the relationship is toxic, *both* people have poor self-esteem and lack personal boundaries.

> It is necessary to understand that healthy people are not in relationships with toxic people. If the relationship is toxic, both people have poor self-esteem and lack personal boundaries.

Toxic people believe, on the surface, that they are good and caring people, and wonder how anyone could leave them. This, of course, is denial at its finest. In their deepest hearts, they are terrified of abandonment and will avoid it at all costs.

Tools for Change

We might wonder if such individuals have a hope of establishing healthy relationships. The answer is yes. However, just as with a chemical addiction, addiction to toxic relationships take people must be willing to see the truth in themselves and to learn and implement new and more effective coping methods. It takes honesty from both partners. Codependents must understand that they themselves are addicted to drama and to the intensity that characterizes codependent relationships. Both partners must learn the difference between the intimacy that is an essential part of honest, healthy relationships, and the intensity of toxic relationships. Both

> Learning the tools for better relationships does not mean life will always be easy. It doesn't mean that we will no longer have differences or arguments with our partners or loved ones. It does mean that we learn to disagree agreeably and respectfully. It means that we learn to give ourselves and others space to grow.

people must learn to communicate in ways that are open, honest, and respectful to themselves and other people.

I do not advocate that anyone stay in an abusive relationship. We are all responsible for our lives and how we live them. I do believe that there are relationships that are too toxic to be saved. However, I have seen many cases in which both partners were truly willing to look at themselves and the parts they played in the relationship—"the dance," if you will—honestly. They did the work of taking responsibility for their own actions and learning to set clear, appropriate boundaries for themselves and their partners. They learned to say, "This is what I will accept, and this is what I won't accept," and, "This is what I will do, and this is what I won't do." In order for the relationship to achieve balance, each partner had to be willing to walk away rather than stay in an abusive, disrespectful situation.

Learning the tools for better relationships does not mean life will always be easy. It doesn't mean that we will no longer have differences or arguments with our partners or loved ones. It does mean that we learn to disagree agreeably and respectfully. It means that we learn to give ourselves and others space to grow. It means that, when we are wrong, we take responsibility and promptly admit it. We learn to say—and mean—the words "I was wrong," "I'm sorry," "Please forgive me," "Thank you," and "I love you."

> We learn to say—and mean—the words "I was wrong," "I'm sorry," "Please forgive me," "Thank you," and "I love you."

CAREY AND SUSAN

Carey was required by the court to seek treatment for alcohol and cocaine addiction and to participate in anger management following an episode in which he slashed his girlfriend, Susan's, tires, kicked down her front door, and wrecked her house. During his initial assessment, Carey explained to me that he and Susan had been at a bar drinking, dancing, and having fun, when a male neighbor of hers sent her a text message asking how she was. Carey said that he felt this was very disrespectful, particularly because Susan did not think the text was a big deal. She told Carey that she was with him, and that if she wanted to be with someone else, she would be. He explained that he felt that if she was his girlfriend, she should not be accepting calls or text messages from "old boyfriends." When he began treatment, Carey was thirty-eight years old and Susan was forty-three years old. Both of them had been previously married and had teenaged children.

Carey went on to explain that, as the argument escalated, he felt the need to confront the neighbor and establish his place in Susan's life. Susan became angry and went home. After Carey confronted the neighbor, who tried to explain that he and Susan were only friends and that he meant no harm, Carey began obsessing about the "relationship" and all the ways in which he felt Susan had been dishonest and disrespectful toward him. He decided to go and confront her, but she did not want to talk to him. In Carey's eyes, this was "unreasonable," even though it was 2 a.m. and he had been drinking all night. He said that all he wanted was for Susan to tell the truth. He became enraged and slashed her tires so that she could not leave. When she wouldn't open the door, he kicked it in. Carey tore through the house, looking for evidence that Susan had been cheating on him.

Susan called the police, and Carey was arrested and charged with domestic violence, public intoxication, and criminal mischief. The judge issued a protective order, stating that Carey was to have no contact with Susan or any of her family members for two years. He was given two years of probation and was ordered to seek counseling for anger management and alcoholism. During the first meeting with his probation officer, Carey violated the orders of his probation by testing positive for cocaine. As a result, he lost his job.

Neither Carey nor Susan followed the protective order, and they continued to text and e-mail each other. Both were in a constant state of anxiety and turmoil. Susan tried to drop the protective order, professing her undying love for Carey and stating that they merely had had a misunderstanding. Both were deeply enmeshed in the drama and toxicity of the relationship, and their consistent, intense fighting continued. The court refused to drop the protective order, and both partners continued to violate the rules.

I explained to Carey that, in order for me to work with him, he must abide by the court requirements. That meant that he needed to focus on his sobriety and honor the rules of the protective order. I told him that he must take the time to look at how his life circumstances were directly related to his belief system and his own behavior. I had him journal his emotions, especially when he felt anger or rage, and write out a plan of action when he felt the need to control other people or situations. This helped him learn to act instead of react when he felt hurt or rejected. I taught him to implement the rule that he could not talk about or act on feelings of anger for three hours after he began having them. This would help him to think, relax, and make better decisions. Above all, he was to abstain from drugs and alcohol in order to clear his thoughts and gain some clarity.

Carey worked hard on learning to restructure his thoughts. He learned to practice deep, conscious breathing in order to slow down his thoughts, his blood pressure, and his heart rate. He attended AA meetings three times a week and came to counseling twice a week. He worked hard on establishing clear and appropriate boundaries in his life. He reported that, at times, he felt anxious and even nauseated when choosing not to react or control other people, especially Susan. When feeling obsessive and struggling with the compulsion to call Susan, he agreed to call his AA sponsor and talk through his feelings.

Next, I had Carey add positive affirmations and a gratitude list to his group of tasks to complete each day. This helped him to improve his self-image and learn to look at the positive aspects of his life.

Carey worked hard on learning more effective coping skills and methods of communication. He learned to sit, listen, and not interrupt when he felt compelled to control a conversation. He learned that listening is the most important aspect of communication and that other people's viewpoints do not have to be wrong for his to be right. He also learned that it is okay to not always be right.

While Carey was in treatment, Susan was also seeing a counselor. She attended Al-Anon meetings and learned to set appropriate boundaries for herself in her relationships. She has learned to see relationships as they are, instead of how she wishes them to be, and to be honest and open with her feelings.

Both Susan and Carey became willing to walk away from the relationship as it was, and Carey has been sober for over two years now.

He and Susan are seeing a therapist together, but have not decided if they want a long-term relationship with one other at this point. They are learning to communicate in a more respectful manner. They have also learned that stressful situations will inevitably arise, and that it is not necessary to overreact to them. Instead, they've learned to implement the coping skills when stressful situations do arise.

Recovery from toxic relationships means identifying and taking down one's masks, learning to be alone, and feeling comfortable in one's own skin. Recovery requires us to dismantle our defense mechanisms and to respect another person's "no." We realize that we don't have to be wrong in order for the other person to be right—and vice versa. We discover that each of our opinions is valid and that we can learn from other people's viewpoints. We understand that we don't have the right to control or change other people. Recovery also means that we do not accept abuse or disrespect from others.

> Recovery from toxic relationships means identifying and taking down one's masks, learning to be alone, and feeling comfortable in one's own skin.

In order to learn to have healthy relationships, people who have been in toxic relationships must come to understand the difference between the two. This means learning to how to be quiet and to listen, and to be teachable. It also means learning to trust our gut instincts and listen to the inner "no." Many people have ended up wounded, or even dead, because they did not listen to an inner voice that said, "This is dangerous—leave now!" Instead, they made excuses for abusers and kept trying to "fix" them. We cannot "fix" other people. We can only establish clear and healthy boundaries for ourselves and be willing to take care of ourselves when other people cross them.

Healthy relationships are based on love, respect, and trust. They are not based on suspicion, anger, or other forms of control. Healthy relationships are based on integrity and appropriate boundaries. Most importantly, they are based on healthy self-esteem.

An important and difficult part of treatment is to identify and dislodge false belief systems and help people see that they can truly be effective in their lives without mind-altering or mood-altering substances, and without having to control other people. Healing from toxic relationships means learning to believe that you do indeed deserve and are capable of having healthy, respectful relationships.

The most important aspect of breaking the cycle of toxic relationships is learning to have healthy, honest, and respectful relationships with ourselves. It is impossible to love others if we do not love ourselves. When people are shame-based in their thinking, the idea of loving themselves seems perhaps arrogant or self-centered. If they grew up in a family that did not foster a sense of self and emotional health, this task will be arduous. Old belief systems will have to be challenged and restructured.

Recovery from toxic relationships takes work. It takes facing deeply ingrained fears and defense mechanisms. It means challenging these self-destructive beliefs and developing healthier coping skills, as well as appropriate emotional, physical, mental, and sexual boundaries. It takes total and complete honesty with others and oneself. It takes open-mindedness and a willingness to live differently.

> True self-esteem comes from the knowledge that we were created in an unbroken, perfect state, and that our life experiences have been for the purpose of nurturing our personal growth and development.

True self-esteem comes from the knowledge that we were created in an unbroken, perfect state, and that our life experiences have been for the purpose of nurturing our personal growth and development.

Some people have a hard time with the idea that they were born perfect, because they have been taught the erroneous concept that they were born in sin—and, therefore, are bad—and that they have to somehow obtain God's forgiveness for this. This idea says that God's creation is less than perfect, and, therefore, God is less than perfect.

Likewise, some people have a very difficult time embracing the idea of a relationship with God. Sometimes this is due to the traumas of their past. Sometimes it is due to family and cultural teachings. Some people are more comfortable viewing God as positive energy rather than as an individual deity.

Just because people do not embrace God in the same ways does not mean that they cannot heal from addictions or other self-destructive thoughts and behaviors. Rather than denying or advocating a specific religion or belief system, holistic methods offer people respect for their individual spiritual beliefs during the recovery process. Holistic treatment offers addicts the tools to develop a personal recovery program that can fit their unique perspectives and grow with them.

> Rather than denying or advocating a specific religion or belief system, holistic methods offer people respect for their individual spiritual beliefs during the recovery process.

4

Addiction to Anger

"For every minute you remain angry, you give up sixty seconds of peace of mind."
—Ralph Waldo Emerson

Our discussion of addiction would be incomplete if we did not address how anger relates to addiction as well as addiction to anger itself. I've devoted a chapter to discussing anger because it is the primary emotion that people recovering from any addiction struggle with. You see, addicted people have been masking or medicating their feelings for a long time; their addictions shield them from emotions they don't want to experience. The object of their addiction has comforted them, and now they have to give up that source of comfort. This can be very frightening and can provoke feelings of anger.

Anger is sometimes referred to as a secondary emotion. It gives us a temporary sense of power or control. In other words, anger is an emotion of self-preservation; it is a reaction to a perceived threat. Sometimes, anger can serve as a powerful motivator to change, to move, to get out of the way of danger, or to leave an unhealthy relationship. Indeed, there are situations in which anger is justified, even necessary. Anger can be a powerful motivator.

However, we must honestly look at our angry behavior. Is our anger hurting those around us? Just as anger can be a motivating factor in our lives, it can also become a toxic way of life and destroy our relationships.

> Ninety-nine percent of the time, our responses to anger remind us of drinking poison.

Ninety-nine percent of the time, our responses to anger remind us of drinking poison. Anger makes us sick, and it hurts us much more than it helps us. It is especially toxic when it *masks* fear or hurt. It is easier for many people to feel anger than to feel the vulnerability of fear or hurt, and this distortion of emotions can have serious consequences.

There are two distinct angles to examine anger from. In some instances, people drink, take drugs, and participate in other self-destructive behaviors because of underlying anger. This type of anger often shows itself as depression, and points to an underlying or core issue.

In other cases, anger can be an addiction in and of itself. When some people have angry acting-out episodes in response to perceived threats, they experience an endorphin release in their brains. This feeling becomes pleasurable. When the behavior is repeated over and over, it becomes people's normal reaction. Anger becomes not a defense mechanism, but their way of being—and their addiction.

We can say that anger is implosive or explosive. Anger that has been masked or medicated falls into the "implosive" category. People who are implosively angry are hard on themselves. Negative self-talk is common for them, and they have poor self-esteem. People with implosive anger are often controlled by others. Implosive anger and depression go hand in hand; in fact, it has been said that depression is simply anger turned inward. We become depressed when we feel we have no choices in our lives, when we feel like victims, and when we are overwhelmed.

People with explosive anger, on the other hand, have a strong need to control and dominate others. In contrast to implosive anger, which is the "flight" part of our natural fight-or-flight response, explosive anger is the ultimate "fight" part of our response. People with this out-of-control "fight" response are hard on those around them and cross other people's boundaries. They display overt anger, which can include hitting, yelling, using profanity, breaking things, reckless driving and so forth.

People with both types of anger lack self-esteem and healthy boundaries.

Anger during Recovery

Many people early in recovery experience very intense feelings. This is because they have hidden their feelings, or avoided their intensity, by medicating them and by developing other defense and coping methods. When they quit using drugs, their feelings seem to be more on the surface.

The intense feelings experienced early in recovery are sometimes due to a chemical imbalance in the brain. Addictive drugs produce similar effects in the brain as our natural neurotransmitters, causing a euphoric feeling or a "high." After repeated use of addictive drugs, the brain's production of neurotransmitters progressively diminishes. The resulting chemical imbalances cause a variety of negative feelings like depression, anxiety, irritability, lack of motivation, fatigue, difficulty concentrating, and so forth.

Sometimes people in early recovery feel sadness and regret due to the losses they have incurred as a result of their addiction. Some people feel deep shame because of their own past behaviors. Many people report an increase in their feelings of anger. This anger comes, in part, from having to give up their source of security: their drug of choice. It has been said that with an addiction, the source of people's sanity is also the source of their insanity.

At the root of much anger is the fear of losing our self-worth. We often base our self-perceptions on what we *think* are others' opinions of us. When we think someone looks down on us or sees us as less capable, we often feel offended. The anger felt here typically masks hurt or fear: hurt that someone thinks poorly of us, or fear that we may be rejected.

Also, when people's needs are consistently unmet, they often live with a deep sense of anger. This makes sense on a basic level: when our essential needs are not met; when we are hungry, tired, overly hot or cold, or in pain, our sense of survival kicks in and we feel angry. We can see this most clearly when we observe babies. Let babies become uncomfortable in any of these areas, and they will most definitely let you know!

Our most basic need in life is the need to love and to be loved. If we do not feel lovable, we will not feel loved. Studies have shown that babies who are not touched, held, and loved have a higher mortality rate than those who are nurtured and feel safe. If we are not nurtured and loved adequately as children, we will grow into adults who feel unloved and unlovable. Many adults who have consistent feelings of anger and discontent feel unloved and unlovable. Because they feel unlovable, they have a very difficult time relating to others and allowing others to be close to them. The very thing they need and want the most is the thing they fear and resist the most.

> Our most basic need in life is the need to love and to be loved. If we do not feel lovable, we will not feel loved.

Explosive Anger

When reactions or responses are repeated over and over, it is as if our brains become hardwired to the response. Some people seem to have a hair-trigger anger response. I refer to this type of anger as an addiction, because it is characterized as obsessive and compulsive, and because it is progressive in nature. People with addictions to anger will engage in angry behaviors regardless of the consequences. Those who live and work with anger addicts will describe them as an angry or resentful. As the angry person's behavior progresses in intensity and frequency, their behavior is not only a reaction to a perceived threat, but it becomes a way of life. Their conversations are about proving themselves right and proving others wrong. They tend to see the world as a bad and dangerous place and think that everyone is out to get them.

In some cases, just as an alcoholic experiences blackouts, a person who rages can experience blackouts. That is, they can't remember what they did or said during a period of anger because they were so angry. These rages are typically followed by periods of extreme exhaustion and depression. Sometimes, people addicted to anger will use the blackout period as an excuse: "If I don't remember it, how can I be responsible for it?"

Treatment methods for these types of individuals can include cognitive behavioral therapy, in which they learn to think about how their behavior affects other people. They must also learn to relate their angry behavior with the negative situations in their own lives. In working with people struggling with anger, I use solution-focused therapy to help anger addicts consider and develop more appropriate methods of communication. I also include deep, conscious breathing, brain-wave synchronization, and meditation in these treatment plans. It is also helpful to teach them to empower themselves with positive affirmations and self-talk.

To repeat, anger can be a mask that people hide behind. Remember, anger is an emotion of self-preservation. The idea of removing the mask can create a great deal of anxiety for people driven by anger. Underneath the masks lies a great deal of vulnerability.

People who are addicted to anger tend to ruminate and spend a great deal of time focusing on the injustices done to them, which increases their anger and resentment. Angry people have higher rates of stress-related diseases, such as hypertension and heart disease. They tend to struggle with substance abuse disorders and related diseases, and have a much higher rate of suicide or accident-related deaths. Many of them experience depression, anxiety, and mood disorders.

Just as dysfunctional behavior is learned, it can be unlearned and replaced with better coping skills. As with any addiction, one of the primary components of anger addiction is denial. Denial of toxic or chronic anger typically comes in the form of minimization or justification. But no matter how people justify their anger, the end result is the same. Chronic anger brings with it fractured and broken relationships, illness, and death.

Tools for Change

So, let's look at how we currently deal with our anger and explore better coping methods.

First, let's go into more detail on the different types of anger responses. When we have an outer, aggressive response to anger, our brains are flooded with endorphins. This is a primal, biological response. Our adrenaline levels rise, our breathing becomes shallow, our blood pressure rises, our vision becomes focused on our adversary, and our body temperature may even change. People who have addictive personalities typically like this feeling, and as mentioned before, that immediate positive payoff is the catalyst for addiction to anger and violence.

We can look at this response and see that it is, indeed, a way of coping with a perceived threat. And, on rare occasions, it is even an appropriate response. However, most of the time, overtly aggressive behavior will create many more problems than it will solve.

Another way of dealing with anger is through covert, or passive, aggression. This inward anger manifests itself in controlling or boundary-violating behaviors that are often underhanded or behind the scenes. Such behaviors include:

- Ignoring the other person.
- Not doing what you say you will do.
- Gossiping and saying hurtful things.

Both overt and covert aggression can be used as a means of getting our way—but they are behaviors that hurt others, not behaviors of integrity. They are ways of dealing with anger, but we can agree there are better, more effective ways of expressing ourselves.

Another way of dealing with anger is suppressing it. When people suppress anger, they typically don't realize they are doing so. They feel they have no power in their relationships, and so expressing their feelings is not acceptable. Many people raised in alcoholic or addicted households learn to suppress their anger. The problem is that unexpressed anger can lead to depression, anxiety, and mood and personality disorders. It can also lead to psychosomatic illnesses, such as rheumatoid arthritis, stomach pain, headaches, and many other physical ailments.

Suppressed anger is like a fire under a pressure cooker that is not properly ventilated: it builds up enough pressure that it eventually blows up. We can all agree that it is not a healthy way to deal with anger.

So, we have to learn to express anger appropriately. In some cases, that means not expressing it at all, especially if we are addicted to anger. I realize this advice seems to run counter to the fact that suppressed anger can have unhealthy effects. But, there's a difference: unlike people who suppress anger and are not in touch with their emotions, people who rage know very well when they are angry—and so does everyone around them.

Because uncontrolled, explosive anger can have long-lasting, multilayered, and devastating consequences, people have to learn to contain their emotions and express them in respectful and responsible manners. This can be a difficult and even painful process for some people. What feel like typical and natural behaviors—sarcasm, finger-pointing, eye rolling, profanity, name-calling, yelling, and violence—must be unlearned and replaced with more appropriate methods of self-expression.

In order to deal with anger effectively, without being either doormats or bulldozers, we must learn to be assertive. Assertive behavior addresses the problem and not the person. It sets appropriate boundaries. It is not about controlling the other person; it is about establishing what we will and won't accept and what we will and won't do. Assertive behavior clearly defines the problem and looks for a solution.

Sometimes the solution may not be what people expect or want it to be. That doesn't mean it is wrong. Assertive behavior does not cross other people's boundaries. It is about accepting responsibility for our own feelings and behaviors, and, if possible, coming up with a solution in which everyone wins. And sometimes, "winning" might not mean what we think it does. For example, if a person wanted to be in a relationship with you, but you didn't want the same thing, then trying to make the relationship happen would be unfair to you and to the other person. In this instance, saying "no" would be the assertive course of action—and it would truly be the most caring way of handling the situation. If you are being true to yourself, you are also being true to the other person in the long run. As another example, let's say you interview for a job, and you find that the job really isn't what you expected or wanted, but you accept it anyway because you need it. Then, six months down the road, you are miserable. You don't enjoy going to work and you don't really give your best effort. Your employer has spent a lot of time, money, and energy training you, and you feel obligated to stay. No one wins in this scenario. Sometimes, "thanks, but no thanks" is the more honest and honorable response.

In some situations, a solution just can't be reached, and we have the choice to drop the topic. This does not mean bringing the topic up during the next fight. It means that we agree to disagree agreeably on this one, or to finally let it go. Painful issues, especially addictions and betrayals, take time and patience to get through. And sometimes. we can't get through them. However, there comes a point when we must forgive and move on with life. Bringing issues up over and over and using them as weapons only brings more pain and hurt into relationships.

If we have chosen to forgive and to stay, we must truly learn to forgive and bring healing to the situation versus anger and judgment. Maybe our loved ones have struggled with addiction and hurt us with inappropriate behavior and words during that time. They have gone to treatment and have made significant changes in their lives. When they are having a bad day, our thoughts return to our own hurt and fear, and we may become accusatory and controlling, bringing up the feelings of the past. Instead, a more loving approach would be to say something like, "It seems you're having a tough day, can I help?" or "I love you and am here for you if you need me." It is not healthy to say, "When you acted this way before, you were about to drink!" or "I don't trust you! What have you been up to?" This sets the stage for defensiveness and closes the door to communication.

So how do we learn to deal with our anger appropriately? The following is a list of coping tools you can learn:

- Check your motive. Are you trying to control the situation or are you trying to bring peace? Be honest with yourself. If you are trying to control or dominate the other person, your motive is based on ego. Appropriate boundaries are about self-care, not "other" control.
- Breathe deeply. This will give you an opportunity to lower your blood pressure, lower your heart rate, and collect your thoughts.
- Pray. Give yourself time to do so. It is very difficult to stay angry with someone you pray for, even yourself.
- Use positive affirmation. Give yourself credit where credit is due. Do the same for the other person.
- Do not view yourself as a victim. When we see ourselves as victims, we remain victims and have no personal power in our lives.
- If you have acted inappropriately, own it and don't make excuses for your bad behavior.

- Apologize. When you apologize, you must mean it, and you must not have expectations about the other person. Do not use apologies as a tool for manipulation.
- Always remember that you, and you alone, are responsible for your thoughts, feelings, and behaviors.
- No one has power over you that you do not give them. When we do not take responsibility for our lives, we are, in effect, victims.
- If anger has created havoc in your life, then be honest about it. You can't change the past, but you can create a better future.
- Take off the mask. It takes courage to put down the mask of anger, but underneath that mask awaits peace, power, and a sound mind.

5

The Healing Process

*"The secret of health for both mind and body is not to mourn
for the past, worry for the future, or anticipate troubles,
but to live in the present moment wisely and earnestly."*
—Buddha

Healing from addiction is a process. It does not happen overnight, and it doesn't happen just by attending a thirty-day program or going to a few meetings. Recovery is about much more than simply abstaining from drugs or alcohol. It means healing from the inside out. It is a true lifestyle change, and encompasses the physical, mental, emotional, and spiritual aspects of people's lives.

Physical Recovery

The first part of this process is physical healing. Depending on the severity of the addiction, this can take some time. While actively addicted,, most people do not take good care of their physical health.

Recovery from every chemical addiction requires a process of detoxification and withdrawal. Chemical addictions are hard on people's bodies and disrupt most aspects of physical health, including our natural circadian rhythms. Our circadian rhythms are the normal sleep-wake cycles that allow for the cyclical release of hormones and the restoration of energy. When we are in balance, our bodies function optimally throughout the day. When these natural cycles are out of balance, we feel tired, irritable, and out of focus.

In order to bring the system back into balance, we have to begin with detoxification, which often involves uncomfortable symptoms referred to as withdrawal symptoms. This process starts when use of the drug stops, and lasts from twenty-four hours to ten days. Detoxification is the physiological or medicinal removal of toxic substances from the human body, during which a person returns to homeostasis, or balance, after long-term use of any addictive substance. The difficulty of the detoxification process is dependent upon the substance involved and people's biological responses.

Once alcoholics or addicts have completed detoxification, they have to do damage control. They need to get their sleep patterns back on natural cycles. Sometimes, people will need additional sleep for a while to recuperate. Natural products, such as melatonin or valerian root, can help to reestablish natural sleep patterns.

It is vital that people in early recovery drink plenty of water in order to cleanse and detoxify the kidneys and liver. Most people who have been using alcohol or drugs excessively are malnourished. It is vital that, as the body heals and returns to natural balance, they eat healthy foods. These foods should include plenty of fresh fruits and green, leafy vegetables, which are rich in antioxidants, vitamins, minerals, enzymes, and other healing agents. It is best to eat a diet rich in fish and chicken and moderate to light in beef. This is because fish is high in essential fatty acids, while beef, although high in B vitamins, is taxing on the body to digest. This is particularly important during the early process, when the digestive organs are healing.

It is important during the recovery process to avoid highly processed foods, especially those high in refined sugar, salt, and white flour. Such refined foods not only provide little nutrients for the body, but they also actually deplete the body of its store of vitamins, minerals, and enzymes; as does the consumption of drugs and alcohol. A healthier approach is to use whole, unrefined foods. Unrefined foods supply our bodies with the basic, raw materials to promote healing.

Another important reason for avoiding highly processed foods, such as sugar and white flour, is that they have a high glycemic index. The glycemic index is a measure of the effects of carbohydrates on blood sugar levels. Simple carbohydrates that break down quickly during digestion and release glucose rapidly into the bloodstream have high glycemic indexes. They include sugar, fruit, sucrose, and alcohol. Complex carbohydrates that break down more slowly, releasing glucose more gradually into the bloodstream, have low glycemic indexes. These include whole-wheat breads, grains, beans, corn, and potatoes; as well as orange and green vegetables.

Eating a diet with a lower glycemic index is particularly important in early recovery. Studies have shown that a high-glycemic-index diet increases cravings in both alcohol and cocaine addicts. Both alcohol and cocaine have very short half-lives. This means they enter the system and leave the system rapidly, creating a craving for more. Simple carbohydrates work the same way. This rapid cycle affects mood and energy levels.

It is very common for alcoholics in the detoxification and post-acute withdrawal phase to crave sugar. This is because alcohol quickly turns to sugar in the body. When the alcohol is taken away, people's glucose levels drop, and they crave sugar. Diabetes and hypoglycemia are common among alcoholics, because the body's ability to metabolize sugar becomes compromised over time. It is wiser and easier on the body during recovery to consume less sugar and simple carbohydrates.

In addition to a healthy diet, we need plenty of exercise. A daily walk outside will not only get your muscles working and your blood circulating, but it will also give you a new perspective on life. People struggling with substance abuse disorders typically have more sedentary lifestyles. As a result, many suffer from both minor aches and pains and more serious chronic pain. Furthermore, abuse of certain addictive chemicals like alcohol can cause the muscles to atrophy. Developing healthy exercise routines is vital in restoring balance to our lives.

In our treatment program, we teach and advocate a yoga practice that not only incorporates basic stretching, but also includes mindfulness, meditation, and martial arts. We consider these practices, as well as exercise in general, to be a fundamental part of our program. Not only is such exercise enjoyable; it also strengthens the body, mind, and soul. It teaches people to get out of their comfort zones and to deal with the stressors of daily living. The practice of yoga and other forms of physical exercise helps to release stagnant energy in the body and builds strength and stamina.

Exercise also improves people's mental and emotional conditions. During exercise, we teach people not to judge themselves; but to train to their fitness level and go just a little bit further. As they see themselves improve week by week, their self-images improve, as do focus and decision-making skills. Many people relate that, after a couple of weeks, they feel the fog lift, and they experience a greater clarity of mind. Exercise increases the release of endorphins in the brain, alleviating the effects of depression, improving anxiety symptoms, and giving people a sense of well-being.

Finally, exercise can improve chronic pain. Many people entering treatment struggle with chronic pain, from migraines to fibromyalgia. Many are withdrawing from opiates. Gentle stretching during yoga; deep, conscious breathing; and mindful meditations are extremely helpful in coping with such discomforts.

Mental Recovery

Alcohol and drug use can have devastating effects on brain functioning. Alcohol destroys brain cells, primarily in the left hemisphere, the seat of language and logic. The number of cells killed varies according to the amount of alcohol consumed. Alcoholics and heavy drinkers kill off about 60,000 more neurons per day than their tee-totaling friends. Renowned psychologist and author, Dr. Pierce Howard states, "Studies of the brains of alcoholic men show reduced blood flow in the frontal lobe, the seat of memory formation, creativity and problem solving." (Pierce J. Howard, *The Owner's Manual for the Brain* [Austin, TX, Bard Press, 2004],, 107)

Howard goes on to cite studies by Ernest Noble, of the UCLA School of Medicine, which show that two to three drinks a day, four days per week, have an adverse effect on brain function, especially in those over forty. My own experiences substantiate these studies; many of my clients have reported compromised short and long-term memory with long-term alcohol abuse.

However, the human body has an amazing ability to heal itself. I have seen positive results in restoring the ability to comprehend and retain information through assigning clients mental exercises. For example, I ask them to complete crosswords or word-find puzzles and read short articles and stories. Exercises that encourage problem solving and memory work well at restoring brain function.

Supplements, including omega-3, omega-6, and ginkgo biloba, have been shown to improve memory functions. The most important vitamin supplements for improving memory are based on vitamins B1, B6, B9, B12, C, and E. The vitamins from the B complex protect the nervous system in several ways. Vitamins B6, B12, and B9 (folate) enhance the memory, and also seem to improve the other mental processes like verbal ability.

Become proactive in your mental recovery. Learning new things, especially complex things like a new language or hobby, is great for improving brain functions, as well as self-esteem.

It is interesting to me that many people with addictions have a natural artistic bent. They are often very talented at drawing, photography, music, or some other form of self-expression. Many times, as their addiction progresses, they quit practicing their arts. I always explore this area with them and give them assignments that get the creative juices flowing again. I am always amazed at the joy people experience when they embrace their passions.

Most of the time, I will assign a book for them to read that encourages personal growth and spiritual development and ask them to share with the group what they learned from it. When people complete the program, they're asked to write a three- to five-page paper about the area in which they have grown the most while in treatment.

Although many addicts are quite intelligent people, they tend to get lost while active in their addictions. Improving mental strength is an important part of the recovery process.

Emotional Recovery

The emotional damage incurred during addiction has two sources. The first is the wreckage of past behaviors and the intense shame that most addicts feel. The second source of emotional damage is the neurochemical imbalance in the brain brought on by the substance abuse.

Addiction is neurological in nature. In an optimum state, neurotransmitters cause the brain to respond appropriately to whatever is happening around us. These neurotransmitters give us a sense of well-being, a sense of alertness, produce pain relief, create a sense of relaxation, and so forth. Psychoactive drugs mimic these neurotransmitters and cause the brain to stop producing them. Whatever the drug does for people, the brain stops doing because it thinks it no longer needs to. When the drug use stops, the brain is no longer producing the neurotransmitters, and people are left with chemical imbalances in their brains. This is why many people entering treatment are struggling with depression, bipolar disorder, and other mood disorders. Sometimes the imbalances are so severe that people may be suicidal or homicidal. In such cases, it may be necessary and appropriate to give antidepressants in order to get the brain functioning correctly again.

Along with psychotropic medications, behavioral changes including yoga; meditation; deep, conscious breathing; guided imagery; self-affirmation; and prayer can greatly improve imbalances in the brain's chemistry. These topics will be discussed in greater detail later.

Above all, in our emotional healing, we must learn to forgive ourselves and forgive others. We must believe in our abilities to heal our lives and in our abilities to connect with other people in loving, healthy ways.

Spiritual Recovery

Spirituality defines our relationships with our highest selves and our relationships with others. The incorporation of holistic healing in the treatment of addictions allows people to develop their own individual spirituality without necessarily embracing a particular form of organized religion. The holistic methods that I advocate encourage people to reach their highest potentials in a lifelong process of personal growth.

> The incorporation of holistic healing in the treatment of addictions allows people to develop their own individual spirituality without necessarily embracing a particular form of organized religion.

Spiritual healing comes from the acquisition of true self-esteem. True self-esteem comes not from what we can get from the world, but from what we can give to the world. Our self-esteem grows when we communicate with the God of our understanding. We do this through acknowledgement and through prayer.

Let's begin by looking at prayer. When we pray, let us pray affirmatively, knowing God's desire for us is good and that prayer coming from a pure heart will indeed manifest abundance in our lives, even if the answer comes in ways we don't always expect or understand.

People recovering from addictions, as well as emotional and physical pain, often find great strength and solace from the prayer of serenity. There is much to be said about repetitive prayers and mantras that serve to focus our minds and hearts. However, sometime we lose sight of the depth of meaning of our prayers when we say them over and over, so it is valuable to go back and contemplate the meanings of what we are saying. As we break down the words of the prayer of serenity, we will see its power and richness.

First we will look at the initial paragraph of the prayer in its entirety, and then we will look at it piece by piece.

God, grant me the serenity to accept the things I cannot change, the courage to change the things I can, and the wisdom to know the difference.

> **God**: The creative life force of all: the energy of love, creativity, acceptance, and abundance.

> **Grant**: To give freely.

> **Me:** The creation and essence of God.

Serenity: Peace of mind, the knowledge that all is as it should be for my greatest good. Serenity comes from a lack of fear. Serenity is a deep, calm abiding in the present moment. I leave serenity when I begin to focus on the past, on resentments, and on regrets. I leave serenity when I leave the present and worry about the future— money, relationships, and circumstances. I return to serenity when I let go of grasping and go back to knowing who I am and where I stand with God and with the universe. I return to serenity when I get out of *"What can I gain from the world or from this person or situation?"* and get back into *"What can I give to the world and to my fellow travelers?"* I return to serenity when I understand that love is the greatest life force and the greatest power in the universe. I return to serenity when I remember that I *am* love in its purest form, as I am made of the essence of God.

Accept: Acceptance knows there are lessons to be learned in each circumstance and that there are always opportunities to grow and to give love—even to myself. Acceptance means understanding that my life is as it should be at this moment. Acceptance allows me to see that sometimes the answer to the question or supplication is "no," and that "no" is indeed the most loving answer at the time. Acceptance allows me to understand the great law of karma, of sowing and reaping. Acceptance allows me to see my fellow travelers from a perspective of love and compassion, rather than with judgment or disdain.

The things I cannot change: There are many things I cannot change, such as the laws of cause and effect. I cannot change the decisions or viewpoints of others. I *can* change my attitude,, and myself, but only when I open my mind and my heart—only when I decrease, so that the Divine Spirit can increase. I can choose to be less rigid and more accepting of the ability of the Spirit of God to work in the hearts and minds of others—even when I don't see it. I can practice acceptance when I understand that my way does not always work, and that God's way always works.

The courage to change the things I can: Courage, here, begins with a non-grasping, non-controlling heart coupled with healthy, life-giving boundaries. Boundaries focus on my behavior, not on the behaviors of others. Boundaries are based on integrity. Integrity means the state of being whole or complete. Healthy boundaries do not allow fear, anger, or judgment of others to control my decisions or perceptions. Healthy boundaries allow love and kindness to govern my life and my relationships with all beings. They also help me to accept other people as being exactly where they are supposed to be on their life paths.

Courage allows me to love others, even when they are not acting lovingly toward me. Courage allows me to see a higher order of life, to stand aside and allow others to walk their paths as necessary, and to have empathy, knowing that God is present even in the most difficult situations.

The wisdom to know the difference: Wisdom gives me the ability to practice what I know to be true. Wisdom understands that *all is well.*

Spiritual healing requires forgiveness of our past experiences and perceived failures, as well as forgiveness of others. When we understand that we are all on paths to become more like the Spirit of God, and that the experiences we have had served to teach us lessons along the way, we can be more compassionate with ourselves and others.

> We must look at our past life experiences and contemplate the lessons we can learn from them. No matter how dark or difficult the situation appears, there is truly a gift in all things if we are but willing to see it.

We must look at our past life experiences and contemplate the lessons we can learn from them. No matter how dark or difficult the situation appears, there is truly a gift in all things if we are but willing to see it.

When we choose forgiveness, we choose to let go of the resentments of the past. Resentments are like weights that hold us down. Resentments keep us stuck and unable to grow. Resentments keep us in the mindset of a victim.

When we choose to forgive, it is for our deepest healing. In the Christian bible, Jesus exhorted us to "forgive others, so that your Father in heaven can forgive you." Jesus knew that, as long as we held on to old hurts and resentments toward others, we would not be free.

6

Alcoholics Anonymous

*"The idea that somehow, someday he will control and
enjoy his drinking is the great obsession of every abnormal
drinker. The persistence of this illusion is astonishing.
Many pursue it into the gates of insanity or death."*
—The Big Book of Alcoholics Anonymous

Bill Wilson and Dr. Bob Smith established the Fellowship of Alcoholics Anonymous in 1935. Thousands of men and women who have participated in Alcoholics Anonymous believe it has saved their lives from the disease of addiction. The program is fundamentally based on the idea that alcoholics understand alcoholics, and therefore can bring a level of nonjudgmental understanding to people struggling with alcoholism.

The Twelve Steps are based on spiritual principles and on the premise that working with a sponsor will help alcoholics awaken spiritually, freeing them from the insanity of compulsive abuse of alcohol and related behaviors. The Twelve Steps are as follows:

Step One: We admitted that we were powerless over alcohol and that our lives had become unmanageable.

Step Two: We came to believe that a power greater than ourselves could restore us to sanity.

Step Three: We made a decision to turn our life and our will over to the care of God, as we understood Him.

Step Four: We made a searching and fearless moral inventory of ourselves.

Step Five: We admitted to God, to ourselves, and to another human being the exact nature of our wrongs.

Step Six: We became ready for God to remove these defects of character.

Step Seven: We humbly asked God to remove our shortcomings.

Step Eight: We made a list of all persons we had harmed, and became willing to make amends to them all.

Step Nine: We made amends to such persons except when to do so would cause them harm.

Step Ten: We continued to take a personal inventory, and when we were wrong we promptly admitted it.

Step Eleven: We sought through prayer and meditation a constant contact with God, as we understood Him, asking only for the knowledge of his will and the power to carry that out.

Step Twelve: Having had a spiritual awakening as a result of these steps we tried to carry these principles to other alcoholics and to practice them in all of our affairs.(2)

(*The Big Book of Alcoholics Anonymous.* 4th ed., [New York: Alcoholics Anonymous World Service, 2002],59-60)

This list can certainly look intimidating, even restrictive, to those who are uncomfortable with the idea of God. For my own part, I must admit that in the beginning, I resisted meetings. I did *not* want to work on those damn steps! No way; I would do it my way, thank you. You see, I've always been a person who's walked to my own drumbeat (one not always within my family's comfort zone). I typically don't accept anything at face value until it makes sense to me. I really did want my life to be better; I just didn't know how to make it better.

It was though reading a wonderful book by Clarissa Pinkola Estees called *Women Who Run with the Wolves* that I found clarity. You see, through my addictions, I had lost sight of my true and authentic self. Dr. Estees is a Jungian psychologist whose work in this book is based on helping women reclaim the wild woman within, the wild woman being their authenticity. I believe the following passage changed my life and set me on a course of reclamation;

> It is these fleeting tastes which come both through beauty as well as loss, that cause us to become so bereft, so agitated, so longing that we must pursue the wildish nature. Then we leap into the forest or into the desert or into the snow and run hard, our eyes scanning the ground, our hearing sharply tuned, searching under, searching over, searching for a clue, a remnant, a sign that she still lives, that we have not lost our chance. And when we pick up her trail, it is typical of women to ride hard to catch up, to clear off the desk, to clear off the relationship, clear out one's mind, turn to a new page, insist on a break, break the rules, stop the world, for we are not going on without her any longer. Once women have lost her and found her again, they will contend to keep her for good. Once they have regained her, they will fight and fight hard to keep her, for with her their creative lives blossom; their relationships gain meaning and depth and health; their cycles of sexuality, creativity,

work and play are re-established; they are no longer the marks for the predation of others; they are entitled equally under the laws of nature to grow and to thrive. Now their end-of-the-day fatigue comes from satisfying work and endeavors, not from being shut up in too small of a mind-set, job, or relationship. They instinctively know when things must die and when things must live; they know how to walk away and they know how to stay.(3)

When I read these words, I underlined them, highlighted them, wrote the word "epiphany," and encircled it with a heart. I knew at this moment that I would do whatever it took to find *me* again, even if that meant Twelve Step meetings! So I went, and I went again. I learned to be quiet and listen. I learned that there was wisdom in those meetings, and I wanted to learn. I got a sponsor. Her name was Lily. Sometimes I loved her, and sometimes I couldn't stand her; but I followed her direction, and I grew.

The Twelve Steps

Let's look at Step One: "We admitted that we were powerless over alcohol and that our lives had become unmanageable." Many people have difficulty with the word "powerless." Some people misunderstand the meaning of this word and mistake it for a sign of weakness. Powerlessness in this context means surrendering to the understanding that we can no longer control alcohol and that it now controls us. I remember the first time I said, "My name is Rhonda, and I am an alcoholic," I thought I would throw up! After all, I was a good little Southern girl, and good little Southern girls were *not* alcoholics. But I knew there was a problem, and I was going to deal with it. Oddly, I felt a sense of peace. Now that I had said it out loud, I could deal with it. It wasn't so powerful, and I didn't feel so ashamed. I still struggle with shame at this point, but I felt safe at those meetings and with Lily.

A thorough understanding of Step One helps us to get out of the denial that has kept us trapped in the insanity of addiction. Denial is the component that keeps people stuck in cycles of self-destruction and life difficulties. Once people can see and understand the severity of their problems, they can begin to do something about it, and their life circumstances begin to improve. Admitting powerlessness is truly an act of courage that allows people to find dignity and rebuild their lives. Working on Step One is the beginning of restoring peace of mind.

> Denial is the component that keeps people stuck in cycles of self-destruction and life difficulties.

An understanding of addiction will help us to see that some people have a chemical reaction to alcohol that does not allow them to control their drinking. Once alcohol enters their systems, the craving for more alcohol takes over. This is much more than the behavioral problem that many people believe it to be. This is why alcoholism is classified as a disease by the American Medical Association.

Step Two says, "We came to believe that a power greater than ourselves could restore us to sanity." The word "insanity" in this context means doing the same thing over and over again and expecting a different result. We may have tried drinking less, starting drinking at different times of day, drinking beer or wine instead of liquor, or some other means of controlling our drinking, only to end up with the same outcome, or worse.

It is at this point that we need someone with some knowledge and understanding—a higher power—to help us see things in a different way. Many people call this higher power "God." . Others have a difficult time with the concept of God. Instead of becoming hung up on this or that perception of God, it is more important to understand that there is a better way to live our lives, and we need to be open to the help of others outside of ourselves in order to recover, feel better, and find some peace of mind.

> Many people call this higher power "God." Others have a difficult time with the concept of God. Instead of becoming hung up on this or that perception of God, it is more important to understand that there is a better way to live our lives, and we need to be open to the help of others outside of ourselves in order to recover, feel better, and find some peace of mind.

Sometimes people understand the love and power of the AA group to be their higher power. Sometimes the higher power is a journal where their deepest fears and secrets are held. Sometimes the sponsor is viewed as a higher power, although a

healthy sponsor will discourage this. I've heard it said that if you can't grasp the idea of God, just accept the idea of good, and start from there.

Step Three says, "We made a decision to turn our life and our will over to the care of God, as we understood Him." Everyone is at a different place on his or her spiritual path. That's okay. What is most significant here is making a decision to get out of self-will—that part of your will that says, *"I want what I want when I want it, and I don't care who gets in the way, I'm going to get it."* It means opening your heart and mind to a new and better way of life, a life with values and integrity.

Step Four says, "We made a searching and fearless moral inventory." Step Four is the step that most people love to hate, and the place where many people get stuck and want to stop! It's frightening to deal with our inner demons—those beliefs and ideas that have created pain and suffering in our lives. What I have discovered over and over is that, when we face those demons, they quickly lose their power over us. By working on the steps, we can even understand that our pasts have served to make us stronger and wiser and helped us to deal with our issues more easily and effectively. Every difficult path we have walked has a gift for us; we just have to see it.

The most important part of life recovery is total and complete honesty with others and with ourselves. In order to change negative behavior patterns, we have to bring them into our awareness. This is where Step Four can help. By looking honestly at our life circumstances and taking responsibility for the roles we played in our problems, we begin to see things differently and relate to others in a more positive way. We learn to have compassion for ourselves as well.

> By working on the steps, we can even understand that our pasts have served to make us stronger and wiser and helped us to deal with our issues more easily and effectively. Every difficult path we have walked has a gift for us; we just have to see it.

As I completed my fourth step, I spent several hours talking to Lily. She gently and kindly listened to every word. She discussed different issues with me and helped me see where I was playing the victim. She helped me to forgive others and myself.

What she said next blew me away. She wanted me to do it again! This time, she wanted me to focus on my toxic relationships with men. This was one of those moments when I went from loving her to not being able to stand her. I moaned and whined; I stomped my foot and argued that it wasn't necessary. She just looked at me lovingly and patiently and said, "I understand, but do you want this or not? Are you willing to do whatever it takes?" I was not happy with her, but deep down, I knew she was right. It was hard. It was embarrassing. Looking at and owning my part in this mess of my life was not easy. She was taking away my right to blame others and be a victim. This was when the real growing began.

It is best to complete your fourth step with a trusted sponsor or even a therapist. Although Step Four can be difficult, it can also be quite freeing and life giving.

What I have learned as a therapist is that, although looking at our character defects during the fourth step is difficult, it is even more difficult for people who are shame-based to acknowledge their character *assets*. Sometimes it is easier to see what's wrong with us than what's right with us. This is why I strongly teach the idea that we were born perfect and good and that those characteristics are still there. The goodness has just been covered up by pain and defense mechanisms.

> What I have learned as a therapist is that, although looking at our character defects during the fourth step is difficult, it is even more difficult for people who are shame-based to acknowledge their character assets. Sometimes it is easier to see what's wrong with us than what's right with us

Step Five says, "We admitted to God, to ourselves, and to another human being the exact nature of our wrongs." It is our deepest, darkest secrets that keep us bound. When we have deep hurts, we either act them out or we talk them out. When we can open up to a trusted friend or sponsor, knowing we will continue to be accepted, these hurts and secrets no longer have power over us. We can face life with renewed strength and courage.

Many people are uncomfortable with this step. They think, *"If I show this person who I truly am, they might not like me,"* or, *"They may see how bad I really am."* The idea of confessing our character defects brings up a great deal of shame and guilt for most people. It is that very shame that

makes us loathe ourselves and keeps us trapped in the endless cycle of addiction.

Keep in mind that your recovery is about you. Recovery is about coming back to a place of wholeness. No one has the right to pass judgment on another person. We have all made mistakes. We have all done things we are not proud of and would just as soon keep secret.

When we can see and accept our shadow side and make friends with it, we begin to see that it doesn't have the power we once thought it did. We must have compassion for ourselves, as well as for others, in order to allow healing in our lives.

> When we can see and accept our shadow side and make friends with it, we begin to see that it doesn't have the power we once thought it did.

As we go through this step, we should bear in mind that our sponsors have also gone through the steps themselves. They understand the fear that this step can create, but they also know the freedom that comes from honestly looking at ourselves, forgiving our pasts, and moving into the present.

Step Six says, "We were ready to have God remove these defects of character." When I first worked through the Twelve Steps, I thought this step seemed silly—wouldn't anyone want God to remove their defects of character? The more I understood, however, the more important I realized this step was. We must be willing to let go of old, self-defeating habits. However, many times we are afraid to do so. We often hold on to our self-destructive behaviors like a dog holds on to an old bone: burying them and digging them back up to chew on them for a while. There is certain comfort in the familiar, even if it isn't good for us.

When we make the decision to heal and to let go of our old defense mechanisms and self-destructive behaviors, it is truly a transformative moment.

Step Seven says, "We humbly asked God to remove our shortcomings." The most important word here is "humbly." Humbleness is when we are no longer in a place of denial or in an attitude of arrogance. It is when we have gratitude for life and respect for ourselves that we connect with a higher goodness.

In my practice, I use two primary tools to help people with this. The first tool is a gratitude list. I ask them to get a journal and write five things they are grateful for every morning. The practice of writing a gratitude list creates a paradigm shift. It's really hard to stay in negative thinking when you're considering what you're grateful for. Other tools I use are letters. I ask my clients to write letters—to God, or to their highest selves. When people are in pain or turmoil, praying becomes very difficult. Writing letters to God helps them to focus on their thoughts and feelings and to get them out. I encourage them not to get hung up on format, spelling, or anything. Just write. If they let it come from the heart, they'll be surprised what comes up. This task has proven to be very healing.

> The practice of writing a gratitude list creates a paradigm shift. It's really hard to stay in negative thinking when you're considering what you're grateful for.

Sometimes, what surfaces is quite painful, and people have a hard time letting go of the past. In these instances, I sometimes perform a ritual with my clients. When people decide it is time to let go, I ask them to write down their memories and painful sensations associated with the past. Then, together, we place the written-down memories in a bowl, and we burn them. I have a beautiful bowl in my office full of ashes in which clients have shared, and then let go of, their most painful secrets with me. When they begin ruminating about the past, we look at the bowl and remember that we have made the decision to let it go.

In this bowl, there are also special treasures including rocks, petrified wood, shells, and other natural items that I have found along my path or that people have offered. Somehow, the beauty of nature has a healing effect. The burning bowl holds a very special place in my office.

Step Eight says, "We made a list of all persons we had harmed and became willing to make amends to them all." It is important to take responsibility for your own actions. Doing so shows maturity and spiritual growth.

Taking responsibility for our lives gives us a sense of self-respect. It takes us out of the victim role. When we decide that our intended course of action is right, and that whatever happens will be okay, we have made a quantum leap into a whole new way of being.

Step Nine says, "We made direct amends to such persons except when to do so would harm them or others." There are certain life situations that prevent us from making amends. However, don't let this be your loophole for avoiding responsibility in uncomfortable situations. If you are in doubt, talk it over with your sponsor. Forgive yourself for the past and move on.

Step Nine is a very healing process, not only for you, but for others as well. Ninety-nine times out of a hundred, when we make amends, the results are positive. Most people have respect for those who have the courage to be honest and to make amends.

Sometimes, those we make amends to are stuck in their own anger and resentments and don't respond the way we would like. That's okay. Say what you need to with an open and pure heart, and accept the response you get with gratitude and humbleness of heart. Sweeping your side of the street is what's important; you can only do your part. Remember, we are all on a path of personal growth in our lives, even if we don't realize it. We must accept and honor others with compassion as they are. Our ability and willingness to do so is a sign of integrity.

Step Ten says, "We continued to take personal inventory and when we were wrong promptly admitted it." Step Ten is about living your life with integrity day by day. It brings transformation and renewal to your life and your relationships on a daily basis. A friend of mine calls this our "daily gut check."

> Step Ten is about living your life with integrity day by day. It brings transformation and renewal to your life and your relationships on a daily basis.

Step Eleven says, "We sought through prayer and meditation to improve our conscious contact with God, as we understood Him, praying only for knowledge of His will and the power to carry that out." Everyone's spirituality is a unique and personal experience. It has been shown over time that, psychologically and physically, people with spiritual foundations heal at higher rates than those who don't.

Spirituality is that place of being at peace with yourself and of reaching out to and caring about others. It is not the same thing as religion, which is defined as the rites, the rules, and the rituals through which people worship.

> It has been shown over time that, psychologically and physically, people with spiritual foundations heal at higher rates than those who don't.

Step Twelve says, "Having had a spiritual awakening as the result of these steps, we tried to carry this message to alcoholics, and to practice these principles in all our affairs." Giving back to others is how we continue to stay sober. Sobriety is a lifelong process. It is an incredible journey that helps us gain insights into ourselves as human beings.

Many people report that working through the Twelve Steps was truly a transforming experience for them. In some cases, people say that the steps saved their lives.

Most people are afraid to go to AA meetings in the beginning. Remember, addicts are ridden with shame in most cases and are afraid that going to meetings will be embarrassing. What makes the fellowship of AA work is that everyone there has experienced the same thing. Different meetings have different personalities, and it's good to try different ones before deciding which one you like the best. Most people feel welcomed and relieved when they go to meetings.

As a counselor, from time to time I hear clients say, "I don't want to hear other people's problems. That can't help me." My experience is that, when people get involved with a Twelve Step group, their chances for achieving successful, ongoing sobriety are much better. Addicts and alcoholics must learn to live differently and must separate from their drug-using friends. AA gives them a new, sober, social support system.

There are Twelve Step groups for many types of obsessive-compulsive behaviors: Alcoholics Anonymous, Narcotics Anonymous, Cocaine Anonymous, Gamblers Anonymous, Overeaters Anonymous, and many others. There are meetings in almost every city in the world, and you can find one morning, noon, or night.

The truth is, the Twelve Steps are the Twelve Steps, and no matter what your drug of choice is, the principles are the same. At one time, many members of AA subscribed to the idea that if people weren't talking about alcohol, they didn't belong there. Fortunately, over time that notion has changed. Many people addicted to alcohol have other addictions as well.

Earlier, I mentioned working with a sponsor. Sponsors are people whom we ask to help us work through the steps. They should be the same gender as us and have a fair amount of time being sober themselves. I suggest someone should have two years of sobriety before becoming a sponsor, but some groups suggest six months or so. Sponsors do not have to be our friends; they just need to be someone we make a connection with. That said, sometimes sponsors do become very close friends in our lives. Their roles are to help us remain accountable and talk through issues and problems that come up.

People will typically announce at meetings that they are willing to sponsor people. Sometimes there is a list of people willing to sponsor others. You may get a sponsor that you don't particularly click with. It's okay to say so and ask someone else. Your recovery is about you and healing your life, so you need someone you feel very comfortable with and who has time to work with you.

The Twelve Promises

The Twelve Promises accompany the Twelve Steps. They affirm that, if we work through the steps thoroughly, certain qualities will manifest in our lives:

> If we are painstaking about this phase of our development, we will be amazed before we are halfway through. We are going to know a new freedom and a new happiness. We will not regret the past nor wish to shut the door on it. We will comprehend the word serenity and we will know peace. No matter how far down the scale we have gone, we will see how our experience can benefit others. That feeling of uselessness and self-pity will disappear. We will lose interest in selfish things and gain interest in our fellows. Self-seeking will slip away. Our whole attitude and outlook upon life will change. Fear of people and of economic insecurity will leave us. We will intuitively know how to handle situations that used to baffle us. We will suddenly realize that God is doing for us what we could not do for ourselves. Are these extravagant promises? We think not. They are being fulfilled among us—sometimes quickly, sometimes slowly. They will always materialize if we work for them.

(*The Big Book of Alcoholic Anonymous*, 3rd ed. [New York: Alcoholics Anonymous World Service, 1976], 83–84)

Al-Anon

Just as addicts have support groups, so do loved ones. Remember, they have taken on their own issues and behaviors and need to deal with those. When couples and families work together, the outcome is often no less than a miracle.

Al-Anon members work through the same Twelve Steps as do alcoholics or addicts. You see, the Twelve Steps really have very little to do with alcohol. Alcohol is only mentioned in the first step. I often tell people to take out the word "alcohol" and replace it with "self-destructive behavior." It will then fit most people.

People who are married to addicts are often adult children of alcoholics. They have carried hurt, pain, and toxic behaviors with them for a very long time. They have to learn to let go of their needs to control everything and everyone around them. Remember, most people who enter treatment do so because their loved ones are looking for peace of mind. Al-Anon is a great place to start.

Just as other Twelve Step meetings can be found morning, noon, and night in most cities; so too can Al-Anon meetings.

7

Healing Neurochemical Imbalances through Holistic Methods

"The art of healing comes from nature, not from the physician. Therefore, the physician must start from nature with an open mind."
—Philipus Aureolus Paracelsus

For many years, alcoholics, addicts, doctors, counselors, researchers, and the loved ones of the afflicted have searched for methods to alleviate the neurological imbalances of addiction. It is the intention of this book to offer techniques that are safe and self-empowering in this ongoing quest. The focus in this chapter, therefore, is to show that controlling brainwave states is a viable alternative for the rehabilitation of addictions and other neurochemical imbalances. Subsequent chapters will focus on *how* to achieve these cognitive changes through lifestyle modifications and methods, such as yoga, meditation, conscious breathing, affirmation, and guided imagery.

The number one need cited by patients entering substance abuse or psychological treatment is peace of mind. This is because when people are active in an addiction or are early in recovery, they often have looping or repetitive thoughts. They are in constant states of anxiety or hyper-vigilance. Many have endured traumas because of their lifestyles. If people have been using psychosomatic drugs, such as stimulants or depressants, for a long period of time, their brain's chemistry becomes imbalanced, as discussed in chapter five. Sometimes, this results in a diagnosis of substance-induced depression or bipolar disorder. Sometimes, people even have psychotic thoughts and behaviors resembling schizophrenia. In such cases, psychotropic medications are often prescribed to relieve these difficult and painful symptoms.

Many clients tell me that they do not want to take medications. I am sometimes amused that clients would drink a fifth of vodka a day or take a handful of pills to get loaded, but refuse psychotropic medications. However, I do understand that by the time they get to treatment, they are tired and truly want to feel what it is like to be clean and sober. Many people report that when taking these medications, they no longer feel like themselves.

My experience has proven time after time that, when people genuinely want to get well and are committed to the necessary lifestyle and behavioral changes, they can heal without the use of psychotropic medications.

The Five Brainwave States

Your brain's nerve cells fire electrical signals that oscillate in distinctive arrangements called brainwave patterns. These patterns are closely connected to your thoughts, emotions, moods, and biological chemistry. Brainwaves are measured using an instrument called an electroencephalogram. There are five different types of brainwaves, measured in Hertz (Hz), or cycles per second. They are associated with different mental states and behaviors. Gamma waves are measured at thirty or more Hz and are associated with high excitement and heightened emotional states. Beta waves are measured between thirteen and thirty Hz and are associated with alertness, anxiousness, concentration, and cognition. Alpha waves are measured at 8–12.9 Hz and are associated with relaxation, visualization, and creativity. Theta waves are measured at 4–7.9 Hz and are associated with meditation, intuition, and memory. Delta waves are associated with detached awareness, healing, and sleep, and are measured at 2–3.9 Hz.

When your body and brain are in optimal emotional, physical, and mental health, these brainwaves synchronize appropriately to the stimuli around you, and your brain produces adequate amounts of neurotransmitters to help you feel alert, relaxed, focused, and peaceful. However, when you are under mental or emotional stress, eating an unbalanced diet, or consuming excessive amounts of caffeine, alcohol, or other mind-altering, mood-altering substances, the natural production of these neurotransmitters becomes unbalanced. Over a period of time, these neurochemical imbalances can result in addiction disorders, depression, anxiety, inability to concentrate, and other mental and physical illnesses.

Stressors

Lifestyle choices other than addiction contribute to neurochemical imbalances. After all, we live in a world today that is constantly on the go. Internet, cell phones, Twitter, Facebook, MySpace, television, and so forth connect us all the time. The common question is, "How much can I get done in the least amount of time?" Because of our ever-advancing technology, our society has indeed gained greater access to knowledge. Through this knowledge, we have a greater understanding of our planet and its inhabitants.

There is, however, a cost to a society that is so fast-paced. The major cost is stress. Stress has been linked to almost every illness of modern society. The list of associated diseases is staggering: heart disease, cancer, high blood pressure, asthma, lupus, rheumatoid arthritis, fibromyalgia … the list goes on and on. And on top of that, there are a host of negative habits associated with the stress response—unhealthy activities people engage in to find artificial relief that include overeating, smoking, and excessive consumption of alcohol.

(Ilchi Lee, *Brain Wave Vibration* [Sedona, AZ: Best Life Media, 2008], 55)

Western medicine tends to treat the symptoms of diseases rather than the causes of them. If we are tired, we take medication to give us energy; if we are anxious or over-stimulated, we take anti-anxiety medications; if we can't concentrate, we take a pill to make us focus; if we are depressed, we take antidepressants. There are times when medication is suggested; however, in many instances, lifestyle and behavioral changes are what we need to regain balance and naturally alleviate the symptoms of

diseases. When we live balanced lifestyles, physical, mental, and emotional health will come naturally.

A balanced lifestyle teaches us to understand the differences between the intensities that typically drive us and the intimacies that give our lives richness and meaning. Balancing our brainwave activities through natural methods gives us the tools necessary to live with meaning and helps create physical, mental, emotional, and spiritual health.

8

Healing with Yoga

*"Yoga, as union, implies perfect harmony
of mind, body and spirit."*
—Sri Kriyananda

*E*astern cultures have long understood yoga as a valuable way to achieve health and well-being of mind, body, and spirit. In *The Yoga Book*, Stephen Sturgess beautifully illustrates this concept:

Yoga, as union, implies perfect harmony of body, mind and spirit. On a physical level, it implies glowing health. On a mental level, it implies the harmonious integration of the personality, and the corresponding elimination of psychological "complexes." On the soul level, yoga implies union of the little self with the greater Self, of ego with the vastness of cosmic awareness, and, as stated earlier, of the individual soul with its infinite source: God. (Stephen Sturgess, *The Yoga Book* [London,Watkins, 2002], xvi)

Healthcare professionals in the West are beginning to see the benefits of yoga as an avenue for healing and as a proactive approach to physical and emotional wellness. Many corporations offer yoga classes to their employees in order to promote environments of health and harmony in the workplace. Research indicates that children and young adults who are taught yoga in schools and on college campuses have a greater ability to focus and retain information, improving their grades, social skills, and emotional wellness. Children derive enormous benefits from yoga. Physically, it enhances their flexibility, strength, coordination, and body awareness. In addition, their concentration and sense of calmness and relaxation improves. Through yoga, children exercise, play, connect more deeply with their inner selves, and develop intimate relationships with the natural world that surrounds them. Yoga brings that marvelous inner light that all children have to the surface.

(Marsha Wenig, "Yoga for Kids," *YogaJournal*, http://www.yogajournal. com/lifestyle/210)

Yoga is used as a viable component of therapy for the treatment of addictive and co-occurring disorders with tremendous success, enabling people to live healthy, productive lives, often without the aid of psychotropic medications. The practice of yoga has become a main component in the treatment of addictions, depression, and other disorders in our intensive outpatient program. Although at times it is met with resistance, when people lean into the practice and begin to see its benefits, they quickly become more open. Part of recovery is learning to get out of our comfort zones and learning to do things differently.

RICK

Rick's story represents one of our successful patient cases using yoga as a component in recovery. Rick entered treatment at our facility in 2006 with a dual diagnosis of poly-substance dependence(addiction to more than one substance), bipolar disorder, and generalized anxiety disorder. This was Rick's sixth treatment episode. His main drug of choice was crack cocaine. He had been arrested for possession of a controlled substance, assault, and for illegal possession of a firearm. He was angry and had been physically abusive to his parents and others.

Rick entered treatment sixty pounds overweight and on a host of psychotropic medications, including a mood stabilizer, an anti-anxiety medication, an antidepressant, and a sleep aid. In prior treatment programs, he was introduced to basic treatment modalities like talk therapy, education, medication, and Twelve Step programs. Although he reported short periods of sobriety and acquired coping skills to deal with his obsessive-compulsive use of drugs, Rick also reported chronic relapse and the inability to maintain employment or successful relationships.

Rick was given a new treatment plan, one that included conscious breathing, meditation, guided imagery, and a healthy diet filled with plenty of fresh fruit, vegetables, and water. He was also encouraged to participate in group therapy, individual counseling and a Twelve Step support group.

While in treatment, Rick was introduced to Dahn yoga. Dahn yoga originated in Korea and is an integrated mind-body training method that combines deep stretching exercises with meditative breathing techniques and energy awareness training. The counselor's goal was to give Rick the tools to help him find the quiet mind and slow down the constant stream of thought that consistently plagued him. This practice resonated deeply with Rick, and his dedication to his recovery and new lifestyle became apparent. He lost seventy pounds in the first six months of practice. His anger was alleviated and he became increasingly peaceful in his demeanor and approach. His need for psychotropic medications lessened as time progressed.

When treatment was completed, Rick remained dedicated to making the practice of Dahn yoga part of his lifestyle. He joined a local yoga studio and furthered his study and practice. Rick now has been sober for two-and-a-half years, is a yoga master, and is working with other recovering addicts. He reports that his obsession to use drugs and alcohol is nonexistent; his relationship with his family is honest, open, and healthy; his self-image is greatly improved; and he feels he has a purpose in life.

JACKIE

Jackie is a forty-six-year-old woman who entered treatment for alcohol and cannabis dependency. She had received a DWI while under the influence of alcohol and then subsequently tested positive for cannabis in a random urine drug screen at her place of employment.

Jackie was required both by the court and her employee-assistance program to seek treatment. She was angry and in denial about the seriousness of her alcohol problem. She was encouraged during her assessment to be open to treatment and just allow herself to learn some new ideas. She indicated that she liked the idea of self-improvement versus the idea of what she viewed as "punitive" treatment.

Jackie's treatment plan included basic chemical dependency education; deep, conscious breathing; meditation; yoga practice; and individual and group therapy. The first two weeks of treatment were difficult for her as she began looking at the belief systems that had led to her current circumstances.

One evening, during yoga practice, while deep breathing and body tapping, Jackie began releasing stagnant, painful energy, and began weeping deeply. Her counselor and her peer group encouraged her to just allow her emotions to come.

The following weeks of treatment were a time of personal exploration and healing for Jackie. Her mood and affect shifted from angry and defensive to positive and peaceful. She began fully participating in all aspects of treatment, and she reported that she no longer craved alcohol or other mood-altering substances. Upon completion of the program, Jackie related that conscious breathing and yoga practice would remain an ongoing part of her personal plan for recovery.

MARK

Mark entered treatment for alcohol dependency. He reported that, along with excessive alcohol consumption, he had started to have anger episodes that were creating problems in his relationships with his wife and children. Mark reported that he was experiencing an overall feeling of discontent and anxiety. He was suffering from insomnia, reporting an average of four hours of sleep per night.

Mark reported, although his primary care physician had encouraged him to take antidepressant and anti-anxiety medications, he chose to take a holistic approach to treatment instead of an allopathic one. Mark's treatment plan included the cessation of alcohol use; plenty of fresh fruits, vegetables, and water; counseling for anger management;

conscious breathing techniques; yoga practice; and Twelve Step recovery meetings.

Mark participated well in all aspects of treatment. His anger episodes began to subside, and he reported improved relationships with his family. Mark became more interested and involved in the practice of yoga, making it a part of his daily routine. His demeanor became more focused and relaxed, and his peers began affectionately referring to him as the "Happy Buddha Guy." When he completed the first phase of treatment, Mark was on no psychotropic medications; he reported that he had been alcohol-free for sixty days, and he was sleeping an average of eight hours per night. When asked to define his relapse prevention plan, Mark reported that he would continue with aftercare meetings, continue eating a healthier diet, and maintain yoga practice as part of his daily routine. Mark has remained clean and sober for ten months, and reports no cravings for alcohol and no anger acting-out episodes.

The practice of yoga has been shown to be effective in helping clients with addictions and co-occurring emotional and mental disorders to regain balance in their lives. Consistent practice improves physical stamina and boosts the immune system. The practice of yoga stabilizes brainwave activity, allowing individuals to solve problems more easily, focus longer, and improve sleep patterns. As people become more balanced in their thoughts and emotional responses, their social interactions improve, as do their relationships with the higher self. Yoga, as a lifestyle, has been shown to enhance self-esteem in those who practice it.

Embracing the calming and spiritual aspects of yoga, including respecting and honoring oneself and others, helps a great deal in developing appropriate boundaries and healthy relationships. The practice of yoga teaches us to calmly lean into the stretch or pose; more generally, it teaches us to "lean" into difficult situations calmly and peacefully.

9

Conscious Breathing: The Cornerstone for Health

"Being aware of your breath forces you into the present moment—the key to all inner transformation."
—Eckhart Tolle

*C*onscious breathing is the cornerstone of emotional, physical, mental, and spiritual health. Deep breathing improves blood circulation, lowers heart rate and blood pressure, and improves strength and endurance. Conscious breathing releases tension and stress and has a profound effect on pain management. Deep, conscious breathing helps us to relax, allowing thought processes to slow down and improving problem-solving abilities. Learning to breathe effectively can create profound improvements in all areas of a person's life.

In his book, *Conscious Breathing*, Gay Hendricks discusses conscious breathing from a spiritual perspective:

In many ancient cultures breath was synonymous with spirit. To the Greeks, spirit was pneuma, the feeling of the breath moving in the body. To the Romans it was spiritus and to the Hindus, atman, the very feeling of God in the body. The enlivening feeling of the moving breath occupies a special place in human experience. Breath is more to us than air: It is life itself, the feeling that lets us know that we are here. In the second chapter of Genesis, God created the first human and breathed into his nostrils the breath of life: and man became a living soul.

(Gay Hendricks, *Conscious Breathing* [New York: Bantam Books, 1995], 73)

Conscious breathing is used in various areas of spiritual practice, including meditation. It allows one to find the quiet mind and opens the heart to a connection with the highest source.

People struggling with addictions need to learn new methods of feeling good without negative side effects. Deep breathing increases oxygen in the body, improving our general health, and that feels good. Deep, conscious breathing gives us the feeling of an organic high—a state that addicts are comfortable with. In early recovery, people often struggle with cravings for whatever substances or behaviors that give them the highs they are seeking. While in a craving state, a person becomes anxious and irritable and moves to beta or gamma brainwave states. Learning to breathe deeply during a period of craving has proven to be very beneficial in alleviating the feelings of anxiousness and stress that accompany the cravings. By focusing on slowing the breath, the client relaxes, moves to an alpha brainwave state, and ceases to focus on the craving. Many clients report that using this coping skill over time often decreases cravings and eventually eliminates them altogether.

It has long been understood that women in childbirth can control their level of pain by using conscious breathing to induce deep relaxation. Deep relaxation induces a generally numb feeling; for example, fewer pregnant women require epidurals during delivery when they practice deep relaxation techniques.

Many people seek treatment because they have become addicted to opiates originally given to them for pain management. These people must learn new methods for controlling chronic pain. Alternative methods of pain management, including relaxation, yoga and deep, conscious breathing, have the effect of releasing natural, pain-relieving endorphins in the brain.

TOM

Tom, a fifty-two-year-old man, came to treatment addicted to alcohol and opiates. He had been diagnosed with a co-occurring condition of major depression and generalized anxiety disorder. He was on antidepressant and anti-anxiety medications. Tom had hepatitis C and cirrhosis of the liver that reduced the functioning of his liver by 80 percent. He was on the waiting list for a liver transplant. He had an ashen, yellow tint to his skin. Tom had chronic back pain and his gross motor functioning was mildly impaired. Any use of alcohol or narcotics would invalidate Tom as a candidate for a transplant.

Although he had few options, Tom was skeptical about alternative methods of pain control, as he had lived with chronic back pain for many years. In order to begin outpatient treatment, Tom's body had to be safely detoxified from alcohol and opiates under medical supervision. When he entered our outpatient treatment program, he had residual, post-acute withdrawal symptoms; including muscle and joint pain, anxiety, and mild nausea.

Tom's treatment plan began with conscious breathing. The treatment team agreed that until he learned deep, conscious breathing, the remaining aspects of his treatment plan would be less effective. Once Tom had a good grasp of conscious breathing techniques, yoga, guided imagery, and nutritional education were added to his treatment plan; as well as individual, group, and family counseling.

Very often, people with chronic pain have to learn how to breathe deeply and effectively. The emotional and physiological effects of chronic pain often result in shallow breathing accompanied by muscle tension and anxiety. Tom approached this aspect of his treatment with an open mind. He occasionally had emotional outbursts and periods of crying.

His counselor explained to him that these episodes were healthy and a normal part of his recovery.

With daily, conscious breathing exercises, Tom, his counselor, and fellow group members began to see significant changes in him. Tom's skin color began to improve and he reported less pain and improved mobility. He began to laugh more and integrate with other group members. Guided imagery helped Tom learn to relax each part of his body individually, and he was taught to "breathe into" his pain. When he became anxious and angry, Tom learned to step back and take ten deep, cleansing breaths before reacting.

Tom eventually had a successful liver transplant. He continued group counseling and also attended a support group for patients who had received liver transplants. He had a brief relapse, abusing pain medication following his surgery. He quickly implemented his coping skills and has now been sober for eighteen months. He continues to attend aftercare meetings on a regular basis. When asked which of the coping ,mechanisms he learned was most important, Tom responds with a smile, "Just breathe!"

Conscious breathing is a viable and necessary coping skill for individuals recovering from addictive disorders and neurochemical imbalances. Conscious breathing teaches clients to slow down their thought processes, alleviating the anxieties that have previously led to obsessive thoughts and compulsive, self-destructive behaviors. These self-destructive behaviors include a relapse of substance abuse, as well as anger and sexual acting-out behaviors. The practice of conscious breathing can quickly move us from a state of confusion, fear, and anger; to a state of peace, power, and a sound mind. If practiced on a regular basis, people are able to remain in this state of peacefulness and equanimity when faced with stressors or difficult life situations.

10

Meditation for the Quiet Mind

"Regular meditation not only restores our inner harmony and vital energy, but provides us with an actual experience of the peace we seek."
—Diane Dreher, The Tao of Inner Peace

Meditation is accepted and recognized by all religious and spiritual practices worldwide. In the practice of meditation, one learns to get in touch with the quiet mind. While prayer is referred to as speaking to God, meditation is sometimes understood as listening to God or to one's higher self. For people in deep emotional pain, meditation can be both a very difficult and deeply healing process.

People active in addictions often report being plagued by tangential thoughts. These clients are unable to focus or concentrate and are often diagnosed with attention deficit disorder. People who have used mind-altering substances often experience intense fluctuations in moods and emotions and commonly meet the diagnostic criterion for depression, bipolar, or other mood disorders.

In the traditional medical model, psychotropic medications are very often part of the treatments for addictions and related disorders. Although these medications can have positive results in the initial alleviation of the symptoms, they are not without unwanted and often dangerous side effects.

The goal of meditation in the treatment of addictions is to teach clients to calm their racing thoughts and get in touch with their true and authentic natures.

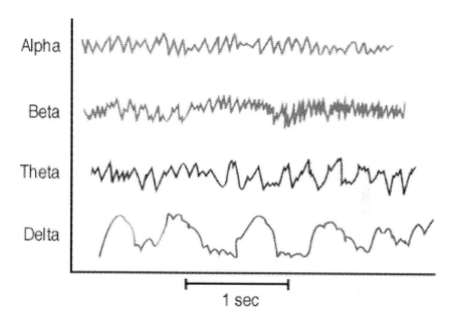

The practice of mindfulness, of bringing the scattered mind home—and in turn bringing the different aspects of our beings into focus—is called "peacefully remaining" or "calm abiding." Calm abiding accomplishes several things: all the fragmented aspects of ourselves, which have been at war, settle, dissolve, and become friends. In that settling, we begin to understand ourselves more, and sometimes even have glimpses of the radiance of our fundamental nature.

(Sogyal Rinpoche, *The Tibetan Book of Living and Dying* [New York: HarperCollins, 1994], 62)

Meditation has been quite successful in relieving the symptoms of depression. It has been shown to synchronize brainwave activity, alleviating the symptoms of attention deficit, bipolar, and other mood disorders. As we slow the brainwave patterns from beta, to alpha, to theta, and to delta, there is a corresponding increase in balance between the two hemispheres of the brain. This more balanced brain state is called brain synchrony or brain synchronization. Through the use of electroencephalographs, it has been shown that the brainwaves of people in deep, meditative states shift from the usual asymmetrical patterns (where one hemisphere is dominant over the other), to a balanced state of whole-brain integration that has the same brainwave frequency throughout.

People who meditate on a regular basis can effectively change the way their brain responds to stimuli that would normally move them to an anxious state or into obsessive, looping thoughts. Instead, they enter an alpha state, in which finding a solution to or acceptance of a problem becomes easier. At first, the effects of meditation are temporary, but with consistent practice, the brain changes over time, creating new neural connections between the two hemispheres of the brain. Gradually, people gain the ability to enter these states at will, even when not meditating, and remain there for increasingly longer periods of time.

Brainwave Entrainment

Brainwave entrainment uses sounds and tones to help people reach a deep state of meditation and relaxation, thereby moving them from an anxious, beta state to a state of alpha, theta, and even delta brainwave states. The goal of brainwave entrainment is to bring the functioning of the two hemispheres of the brain into balance. When the brain is out of balance, people are in a state called brain lateralization, in which they see and experience themselves as separate from and in opposition to the rest of the world. In his book, *Thresholds of the Mind*, Bill Harris explains brain lateralization:

The greater the lateralization in the brain, the greater the feelings of separation—and the greater the feelings of separation, the greater the fear, stress, anxiety and isolation. In its extreme form, a lateralized, unbalanced brain results in behavior commonly described as dysfunctional or addictive, with all the painful experiences that accompany that state.

(Bill Harris, *Thresholds of the Mind* [Beaverton, OR: Centerpointe Research Institute], 2007)

Traditionally, meditation is practiced by focusing on an object, event, or thought; be it a prayer, mantra, the breath, or a candle flame. These methods of meditation do work to alleviate the effects of brain lateralization and to improve one's quality of life. Any kind of focus will bring about a degree of brain synchronization. This ability to stay in slower brainwave states, however, can take time, sometimes years and even decades, to perfect. It can take even longer for these states to have a lasting effect.

Brainwave entrainment refers to the brain's electrical response to rhythmic sensory stimulation, such as pulses of sound or light. When the brain is presented with a rhythmic stimulus, for example a drumbeat, the rhythm is reproduced in the brain in the form of electrical impulses. If the rhythm becomes fast and consistent enough, it can start to resemble the natural internal rhythms of the brain: brainwaves. When this happens, the brain responds by synchronizing its own electric cycles to that rhythm. The uses of audio recordings that mix embedded, binaural beats with music or various background, sounds are diverse. These recordings can promote relaxation, meditation, stress reduction, pain management, improved sleep quality, decreases in sleep requirements, enhanced creativity, learning, and intuition. Audio recordings embedded with binaural beats are often combined with various meditation techniques, as well as positive affirmations and visualizations. In my experience, this technique has worked very well in the areas of stress reduction, pain management, and improved sleep quality. I have witnessed positive outcomes using brainwave entrainment for these issues. It would stand to reason that, with a relaxed mind, intuition, creativity, and learning ability would improve; however, I do not have documented case studies. I look forward to further research in these particular areas.

Medicine men and shamans of antiquity practiced brainwave entrainment, although they didn't use that term. They understood that a trance state could be achieved through a rhythmic drumbeat. Our ancestors used the practice to prepare the mood of warriors readying for battle or a great hunt. In fact, the drumbeat has been used in all kinds of ceremonies, from bringing rain to celebrating rites of passage. Many of us have experienced dramatic mood changes by listening to classical composers such as Bach and Beethoven. We feel nostalgic when we hear the music of our adolescence. The subtle difference is that brainwave entrainment forces the brain into specific synchronization in order to affect certain outcomes, such as relaxation, stress management, or pain reduction. It can help synchronize brain patterns to encourage the natural circadian rhythms of the sleep cycle.

Likewise, Dahn yoga uses rhythmic music to encourage people to focus on their brain stems and enter trancelike states. They are then encouraged to naturally move whatever parts of their bodies that are necessary for healing, trusting the wisdom of the brain and body to know what it needs. This practice is not only fun; it also releases neurochemicals in the brain that calm and relax.

Both methods of meditation—brainwave entrainment and traditional meditation—can be very effective, depending on people's goals. Traditional meditation involves ritual and puts one in touch with the quiet mind and the higher self. As a life practice, traditional methods of meditation are enriching and life-giving but require self-discipline and time to achieve significant results. The use of brainwave entrainment programs, such as the Holosync Solution by Bill Harris of the Centerpointe Research Institute, can help acutely suffering clients quickly synchronize their brainwaves. This can allow clients to bypass the use of psychotropic medications in the treatment of anxiety, depression, and mood disorders.

Because the Holosync Solution and other such programs have such rapid effects, many clients report that deep emotions, anxieties, and repressed memories of unresolved traumas sometimes surface. Clients are encouraged to work through these feelings using conscious breathing and talk therapy with a counselor or life coach. As people's brainwave states begin to synchronize and they experience an alpha state more often, issues that presented themselves as anxieties or problems take on the quality of questions to be answered.

ANDREW

Andrew presented for treatment with an addiction to sedative hypnotics. He had developed such a tolerance to these medications that he was taking several pills at a time throughout the day in order to relax and cope with the demands of a stressful job as an oil field sales consultant. As Andrew's addiction progressed, his brain's chemistry became imbalanced. He reported that he was unable to sleep and that he had become irritable and aggressive with his clients and his associates. His behavior resulted in the loss of his job. He was unable to maintain his living expenses and had to move in with his elderly parents. In order to support his addiction, Andrew began stealing money from his parents and close friends.

Before Andrew was admitted for treatment, he had to be safely detoxified with medical supervision and protocol. He was admitted to our intensive outpatient program three days later. His treatment plan upon admittance included but was not limited to the use of brainwave entrainment.

Andrew's counselor worked with him daily using deep, conscious breathing and other relaxation techniques that included guided imagery and yoga. For two weeks, he was encouraged to use headphones and listen to a CD created with binaural beats that took him into an alpha brainwave state and then to a theta brainwave state for thirty minutes each day. Andrew reported feeling very relaxed and balanced during the process, but the feeling of relaxation did not last for long periods of time. The third week, his meditation was increased to one hour a day and he began using a CD that induced delta brainwave states, taking him into a deeper state of relaxation. He reported that he was sleeping better and had fewer episodes of anxiety.

After eight weeks, Andrew reported feeling more balanced. He was sleeping uninterruptedly for seven to eight hours each night. He was stepped down to a supportive outpatient program, where he continues to work on implementing coping methods to help him deal with the stressors of his daily life. With his brainwave activity in a more balanced state, Andrew is better equipped to use the neocortex and limbic systems of his brain in problem solving and appropriate decision making, improving his relationships with his family and friends.

When the brain is active in an addiction and in a constant state of beta or gamma, clients rely on what is referred to as the reptilian, or reactionary, part of the brain. When in a constant state of anxiousness, people have more obsessive and compulsive thinking, thus driving addictive behaviors. Controlling brainwave states through the use of traditional meditation, or through the use of sounds and tones, is a viable treatment for neurochemical imbalances.

Treatment that includes meditation and brainwave entrainment will bring to the surface the shadow aspects of people's personalities, resulting in feelings of shame and guilt. I have found that I need to be prepared to help clients navigate through these feelings of anxiety and come to a place of forgiveness of self and others. During the practice of meditation, clients learn to witness these thoughts without judgment, thus finding a sense of peace and acceptance.

Although I think brainwave entrainment is a viable, complementary approach in the treatment of addictions and neurochemical imbalances, it does not replace the practice of mindful meditation. Meditation teaches one to find the quiet mind, which is often foreign to addicts who are always trying to alter their emotional states. With practice, meditation encourages us to become comfortable with ourselves. It teaches us that within the recesses of our minds lie the answers to all of our emotional and spiritual afflictions.

11

Guided Imagery

"You need not wrestle for your good. Your good flows to you most easily when you are relaxed, open, and trusting."
—Alan Cohen

*M*any people suffering from addictive disorders or neurochemical imbalances cannot relax physically, mentally, or emotionally. This constant state of hyper-vigilance is due in part to imbalances of neurochemicals, like serotonin, dopamine, and norepinephrine in their brains. The cause of these imbalances is sometimes hereditary. Addiction disorders, depression, bipolar disorder, and schizophrenia can all be genetically passed from one generation to the next.

Neurochemical imbalances can also be the result of unresolved traumas or the recurrence of traumas in one's lifestyle. For instance, if children are raised in tumultuous, alcoholic, or abusive families, they learn particular coping behaviors in order to deal with the turmoil. These behaviors may include isolation, anger responses, or even panic. Children may go from states of relaxation to states of anxiety or stress, never knowing what to expect from their caretakers. They will often develop obsessive-compulsive behaviors as they try to create order in a confused environment. Any of these coping behaviors, repeated habitually over a period of time, will negatively rewire how the brain responds to stress.

Guided imagery, sometimes referred to as guided meditation, is a powerful tool to help clients change their responsive behaviors. Guided imagery can help people move from anxious, beta brainwave states to more relaxed alpha and even theta states.

There are many forms of guided imagery that help people in a variety of ways. The body scan is a form of guided meditation that encourages people to visualize and relax each part of their bodies. The guide instructs clients to begin by closing their eyes and practicing deep, conscious breathing. The guide then teaches them to focus on and breathe into the toes, feet, ankles, and so forth, working their way throughout the entire body. Clients are encouraged to relax each part of the body and enter into a state of calm abiding. This form of guided imagery is helpful in the relief of stress and insomnia.

> Just as the physical body has a system of interrelated organs, a person's "energy body" has a system of interrelated organs called chakras. When these energy bodies are out of balance, so are our moods.

Another form of guided imagery is chakra balancing. Just as the physical body has a system of interrelated organs, a person's "energy body" has a system of interrelated organs called chakras. When these energy bodies are out of balance, so are our moods.

In his book, *Chakra Therapy*, Keith Sherwood explains:

> When any of the chakras or organs of the subtle energy system are disrupted or damaged, a particular subfield is disrupted, energy becomes blocked, its frequency is distorted and the subfields become contracted. These blockages and disturbances are transmuted to neighboring subfields affecting them negatively and causing them to contract as well. These disruptions are the root cause of all forms of mental, emotional and physical disorders.
> (Keith Sherwood, *Chakra Therapy* ;[St. Paul, MN: Llewelynn, 2002], 5–6)

Chakra balancing begins with deep, conscious breathing. Clients may stand in a relaxed position, lie down, or sit in a half-lotus pose. When breathing is regulated, attention is brought to the first chakra, located at the base of the spine. This chakra represents our rootedness and connection to the earth. Clients visualize the chakra as a red light gently working its way up the spine to the brain's stem. Clients are encouraged to continue deep breathing; visualizing healing, cosmic energy entering into this area on the inhale and releasing stagnant, stressful energy on the exhale.

The attention is then brought to the second chakra, located in the pelvic area. This chakra represents our passions, desires, and creativity. Clients visualize this chakra as orange and are encouraged to breathe cosmic energy into this area on the inhale, releasing stagnant, stressful energy on the exhale. This procedure continues in the same manner, guiding clients through all seven energy organs. Chakra balancing is healing to the mind, body, and spirit.

Another form of imagery that must be guided by a therapist or skilled practitioner is reliving a traumatic incident through hypnosis. The purpose is to release the hold the traumatic experience has on the individual. When people experience trauma, the fear, pain, and anxiety become stuck in their bodies, especially in the chakra system. In some cases, clients suppress the most difficult aspects of the incident. In many cases, they will develop unhealthy coping skills in an attempt to manage the anxiety surrounding the incident. These attempts at coping may include drinking, drug abuse, sexual or anger acting out, obsessive-compulsive behaviors, or panic. People remain in constant beta or gamma brainwave states. Sleep and eating patterns become interrupted, and the overall tasks of daily living become difficult.

The longer people remain in this state without intervention, the more their lives are disrupted and the more the destructive coping behaviors are cemented. When clients relive incidents through guided imagery, they experience, and talk about the incident, and the power of the memory diminishes. In time, people's brainwave states return to their natural cycles, appropriate to the stimuli of their environments.

SHELLEY

Shelley, a nineteen-year-old woman, was admitted to treatment for alcoholism and generalized anxiety disorder. She had been given a diagnosis of post-traumatic stress disorder following a rape incident that had occurred six months prior to admittance. She reported that her drinking had increased substantially following the trauma, and she was plagued with panic attacks on a daily basis.

Shelley reported that she was unable to attend college because of her panic attacks, and that her relationship with her parents was strained as a result of her drinking and rages. She was on antidepressants and an anti-anxiety medication. She was also prescribed Camprall, a medication to help control her alcohol cravings.

Shelley's treatment plan included an intensive outpatient program, yoga, deep, conscious breathing, and journaling. She also attended individual sessions with her counselor in which she participated in guided imagery that included reliving the incident. This procedure was practiced daily for a week. In each session, Shelley was able to emote, or fully experience and express, her feelings of anger, fear, and anxiety. Her initial sessions were filled with periods of crying, anger, and deep grief. By the end of the first week, the intensity of her emotions lessened.

Shelley was then taught chakra balancing and instructed to practice it on her own daily. This helped Shelley learn to bring herself back into natural harmony. She was encouraged to journal her progress so she could track herself and note her improvement.

Shelley was also taught the body scan as a method of relaxation. This gave her the tools to bring herself back to an alpha wave state, where she could manage her feelings of panic and anxiety and problem-solve more effectively.

Shelley participated well in all aspects of her treatment. She is no longer on anti-anxiety medication or medication to control her cravings for alcohol. Her relationship with her parents has been restored with trust and healthy boundaries. She has been sober for eighteen months and recently completed her second year of college with a 4.0 grade point average. She continues to participate in individual counseling as needed and attends aftercare meetings on a weekly basis.

Guided imagery is a very powerful tool in the treatment of addictive and neurochemical imbalances. It gives clients self-empowering thoughts, enabling them to bring themselves from a state of anxiety and confusion to one of alpha brainwave activity, where problem solving and rational thought become easier. With this powerful tool, clients are able to achieve success in ongoing recovery without experiencing painful relapses into old behaviors.

With practice and skill, guided imagery is a creative and effective way for individuals to reach the deeper recesses of the mind, the theta brainwave state. They can begin to sort through and make sense of conflicts and self-destructive behaviors. They can begin to rediscover and rely on natural intuition where appropriate, and make effective decisions.

12

The Power of Affirmation

*"Whatever the mind of man can conceive
and believe, it can achieve."*
—Napoleon Hill

To change our behaviors, we must change our thinking. All dysfunctional behaviors result from faulty beliefs about the self. If we believe ourselves to be hopeless or helpless, then we are. If we believe ourselves to be capable and powerful, then we will be.

Webster's Encyclopedic Dictionary defines *to affirm* as "to state positively, with conviction; to make a declaration of truthfulness; to make a statement of the affirmative (as opposed to the negative)." Affirmations are used to help us complete an action or reach a goal. When we affirm a thought or an idea, we seat them into our belief systems.

> All dysfunctional behaviors result from faulty beliefs about the self.

Many clients enter treatment believing that they are victims of their diseases, their pasts, their family of origin, lost lovers, and so on. Most believe that they are incapable of healing themselves. Affirmations work wonderfully to dispel these ineffective and false beliefs and to reestablish new, effective beliefs.

If people tell themselves that they're going crazy, will be hurt, or will fail, then they become entrenched in beta or gamma brainwave states. In these states, people become anxious and fearful. They have a very difficult time trusting themselves or others. Affirmations can help counteract the vicious self-talk that keeps people stuck in this loop of negativity.

Affirmation is another means of rediscovering serenity. The primary purpose of an affirmation is not to change objective reality, but to change subjective reality. What that means is that we are changing the inner material: our attitudes and thoughts about our relationships, and our approaches to activities and our ways of life.

(Emmett E. Miller, *Deep Healing* [Carlsbad, CA: Hay House, 2008], 107)

This means we are changing our relationship to the circumstances in our lives, not the circumstances themselves.

This idea works particularly well for those dealing with anger and rage. They believe that rage is the only option they have; their brains are wired to react in inappropriate and controlling ways when things don't go the way they want or expect. They know their behaviors are wreaking havoc in their relationships, but they don't have the skills to do things differently. They have been patterned this way from childhood. With the use of affirmations, people are able to move from beta or gamma states to an alpha state, where they can choose more appropriate and effective behaviors.

ROBERT

Robert, a fifty-year-old man, entered treatment for anger and rage problems. A recovering alcoholic, he was never given the tools to deal with his anger. Robert reported that he had struggled with raging episodes since he was a child, and that when he raged, he had blackouts, or periods in which he didn't even remember what he'd said or done. He reported that his wife and children became afraid of him and retreated when he was in a "mood."

Robert explained that he felt deep shame and remorse following anger episodes, and wanted desperately to handle himself with integrity.

Robert's treatment plan included individual, group, and family counseling. He was taught several coping skills to deal with his anger, including deep, conscious breathing; relaxation techniques; chakra balancing; and positive affirmations. Robert related that, of all the skills he was taught, the ones that were most effective and that he used the most were affirmations such as:

- *"I can cope. I don't have to get angry."*
- *"This is only a hassle. I can handle hassles."*
- *"I can control my emotions. They don't control me."*
- *Breathe!"*
- *"Bring water to the fire, not oil."*
- *"Stop, look, listen, think, and then act."*
- *"I will stay in integrity—no matter what."*

Robert reported that when he used affirmations, his mind relaxed, and he was able to think and act appropriately. Robert attended individual, group, and family counseling for one year. He now continues to attend family sessions and teaches anger-management skills to his weekly aftercare group. His self-image has improved a great deal. His relationship with his wife and children has also improved as they have learned effective communication skills and appropriate boundaries.

Positive affirmations help us to get back in touch with our true and authentic selves. They have the power to help us see ourselves from a perspective of integrity and wholeness. Affirmations serve to give us back our dignity and self-respect.

Although affirmations are generally used in a positive manner, they can also be used in a negative manner. Negative affirmations can reinforce impaired self-image, depression, and poor mental functioning. In these cases, we have to look at errors in thinking and logic and come up with new and positive thinking that empowers us to heal these deep-rooted beliefs. Examples of negative affirmations are:

- *"I knew this would go badly. It always does."*
- *"I don't deserve to be happy."*
- *"I'm an idiot!"*
- *"Nothing ever works out for me."*

- *"I don't do anything right."*

It is important to understand that our thoughts are extremely powerful and create the outcomes in our lives. If we believe ourselves to be hopeless, undeserving, and unable, that is exactly what we will manifest. If we believe ourselves to be capable, deserving, and powerful, we will be.

Healthcare professionals must consider teaching wellness practices to patients seeking treatment for addictions and co-occurring disorders. Although there are cases when an allopathic approach to treatment is indicated, such treatment should be reserved for severe cases of depression and psychosis. When practitioners offer a pill for any feeling of discomfort, they merely reinforce escapism. Instead, patients need to learn how to "lean" into their discomfort and accept that life offers all emotions, including sadness, anger, boredom, peacefulness, and joy. This empowers them to live full and authentic lives; to experience and develop deep, meaningful relationships with themselves and others.

Through the use of our inner strengths and beliefs, we are able to heal almost all emotional, mental, and spiritual maladies. The practice of yoga; deep, conscious breathing; meditation; guided imagery; and affirmations helps us to control our brainwave states, thereby healing ourselves of addictive and neurochemical imbalances. Ultimately, we are able to bring our lives back into balance and establish or reestablish cycles of mental, emotional, and physical health.

13

Auricular Acupuncture

"We expected acupuncture to improve pain. We didn't really expect the largest benefit to be in fatigue or anxiety."
—David Martin, MD

*A*cupuncture is a Chinese medicinal art that has been around for centuries and has been used to successfully alleviate physical, mental and emotional ailments of all kinds. Acupuncture is time-tested and is a proven, evidence-based method of treatment.

A report from a Consensus Development Conference on Acupuncture held at the National Institutes of Health (NIH) in 1997 stated that acupuncture is being "widely" practiced by thousands of physicians, dentists, acupuncturists, and other practitioners for relief or prevention of pain and for various other health conditions. According to the 2002 National Health Interview Survey, the largest and most comprehensive survey of complementary and alternative medicine (CAM) used by American adults to date, an estimated 8.2 million US adults had used acupuncture in their lifetime, and an estimated 2.1 million American adults had used acupuncture in the previous year.

Auricular acupuncture is a widely used microsystem within Ancient Eastern Medicine. Microsystems use one area, or aspect of the body—for example, the ears, hands, or feet—to treat conditions that can be present anywhere in the body.

Auricular acupuncture can help with alcohol and drug addiction rehabilitation. When used in the treatment setting during the acute detoxification phase, acupuncture is very effective in alleviating nausea, pain, and anxiety commonly associated with withdrawal. Acupuncture helps patients become more comfortable and focused in their treatment process and stay engaged in treatment longer. One of the main reasons people quit treatment or return to their drug of choice is to alleviate physical or emotional discomfort. Acupuncture helps relieve this discomfort.

When a person is going through the initial withdrawal stage from alcohol and drug addition, it is important for them to receive an acupuncture treatment daily until they are able to be abstinent from drugs and alcohol. Once the person is feeling better and has ceased their usage of drugs and alcohol, the frequency of acupuncture treatments can be decreased to once or twice per week for several weeks. It is recommended that acupuncture treatments continue on a monthly basis for the recovering person. This helps to maintain balance, calm, and focus.

When combined with psychological counseling with addiction specialists and participation in recovery support groups, acupuncture can be a very effective complementary practice in a person's recovery program. Not only does acupuncture work well in the acute stage of detoxification, acupuncture helps manage post-acute withdrawal symptoms, such as anxiety and depression, and helps the recovering person manage cravings. In my practice, I use the National Acupuncture Detoxification Association (NADA) protocol for auricular acupuncture extensively with my clients. The NADA protocol uses five specific ear acupuncture points on each ear for addiction treatment:

Sympathetic point – Balances sympathetic and parasympathetic nervous systems and has a strong analgesic effect.

Shen-men point – Called "Spirit Gate," has a calming and relaxing effect to help alleviate anxiety and nervousness that can accompany withdrawal.

Kidney point – Tones and stimulates the source of energy and essence that is often damaged through chemical abuse. The kidney point can also help resolve fear and increase the willpower needed to overcome addiction.

Liver point – Stimulating the liver point promotes repair of the liver from drug and alcohol abuse and aids in resolving anger and aggression.

Lung point – Strengthens the immune system and accelerates detoxification. Emotionally, it is associated with grief and letting go.

In the mid-1970s, Michael Smith, a medical doctor at Lincoln Hospital in the South Bronx area of New York, modified an existing system of auricular acupuncture into a simple technique for the treatment of many common drug addictions. He did this as an alternative to using methadone for the treatment of opiate addiction. This selection of ear points proved to be extremely effective in the treatment of addictions and became what is now referred to as the NADA protocol.

The original NADA protocol consisted of electrical stimulation on the lung point of a patient's ear. It was soon discovered, however, that inserting tiny needles into the same point produced a more prolonged effect than that produced by electric stimulation. Gradually, adding Shen-men, a well-known ear point that produces a sensation of relaxation, expanded the protocol. Over the next few years, other points were added based on pain resistance, sensitivity, and other clinical factors. The NADA protocol used today consists of the insertion of small, stainless steel, disposable acupuncture needles into five points on the outer surface of a person's ear. The points used in the NADA protocol are sympathetic, Shen-men, kidney, liver, and lung.

In a typical session, both ears are stimulated, or needled, at the same time, usually for between thirty and forty five minutes. Sometimes the procedure is done in an individual setting other times, in a group setting. When acupuncture is done in a group setting, it helps build support among those being treated and helps break down feelings of isolation and fear. I have found both methods of treatment very effective.

My clients have reported that auricular acupuncture is comfortable and enjoyable. In many cases, they report that they have less anxiety and discomfort and are more focused in their treatment and recovery process.

So, how does it work? The effectiveness of acupuncture is certain, but exactly how it works is a mystery. Acupuncture is an Eastern medicine treatment in which acupuncture needles are inserted into the body. The needles are inserted into acupuncture points to adjust the Qi (pronounced chi), or energy, of our body. These acupuncture points exist along energy channels called acupuncture meridians, which connect the surface of our body with our internal organs. By altering the flow of Qi, acupuncture can help people naturally detoxify from addiction and substance abuse. People treated with auricular acupuncture often report an improved sense of balance and calm. Clients often state that they feel "energized," "lighter," and "more relaxed" after undergoing a session. In most cases, they request more follow-up sessions following the initial treatment because they feel so relaxed and peaceful. In addition, they report that the effects last for several hours—even several days, in some instances.

JANA

Jana came to treatment for alcoholism after her husband of thirty years filed for divorce. She reported that she had been in treatment numerous times and had never been successful for any length of time. She was suffering from anxiety and depression and reported a great deal of anger and resentment.

Jana agreed to try acupuncture as an adjunct to her treatment plan, which included daily Twelve Step meetings, yoga, deep conscious breathing and individual solution focus talk therapy. During the first week of treatment, she was given a forty-minute acupuncture session each day. Jana reported a general feeling of relaxation and reduced anxiety. We also included yoga and deep, conscious breathing for two, hour-long sessions during the initial week of treatment.

The second week of treatment repeated the same protocol, and Jana reported that not only was she less anxious; her sleep patterns had improved and she was more focused. She reported that she was better able to participate in her Twelve Step meetings and therapy sessions with her counselor. During the third through eighth weeks of her treatment program, we reduced acupuncture treatments to three times per week.

After she completed the initial phase of treatment successfully, Jana then continued to attend Twelve Step meetings three times a week. She continued acupuncture twice weekly for six months and had weekly sessions with her counselor to address her feelings of grief and loss following her divorce and to develop appropriate coping methods to deal with her anger and anxiety. Jana has remained sober for eighteen months. She continues acupuncture on a bi-weekly basis. Jana reports that although she has some difficult days, her depression and anxiety have been greatly reduced without the use of prescribed anti-anxiety and antidepressant medications. She reports very minimal cravings and says she has developed coping skills through working with her Twelve Step sponsor and her therapist.

Not only is acupuncture effective in working with addictions, I have found that using auricular acupuncture is a very effective tool in helping people who have been injured or traumatized and are suffering from post-traumatic stress disorder. Many people report that they are able to relax and become more "present" in their therapy process. The relaxation achieved through the combination of deep, conscious breathing and acupuncture helps release the tension and fear associated with trauma, enabling the person to work through the trauma and accelerate healing.

MARIA

Maria is a fifty-five-year-old Hispanic female who was referred to counseling by her chiropractor for pain and anxiety following an automobile accident in which she and her husband were hit broadside by another vehicle. Maria reported anxiety every time she rode in a car. She related that she dreamed about the accident nightly, had bouts of crying throughout the day, and was suffering from muscle aches and back pain.

I treated Maria with a forty-minute acupuncture session daily for the first two weeks. This helped her relax enough to learn the body scan technique and participate in deep, conscious breathing exercises. The body scan is a technique in which the person focuses on each area of the body. The aim is to train the person to focus while remaining mindful and accepting toward any sensation that may arise. In the case of pain and muscle tension, science shows that accepting sensations is more effective than trying to control them. Maria was unable to participate in talk therapy at this point. As treatment progressed, we continued acupuncture three times a week and added solution-focused talk therapy, where Maria was able to discuss the accident and her fear of riding in the car with her husband. We began each therapy session with a thirty-minute acupuncture session. When Maria retold the story of the accident she began crying, releasing the effects of the trauma. After a month of acupuncture and talk therapy combined with gentle yoga stretches and deep breathing, along with continued work with her chiropractor, Maria reported that she was sleeping better and the accident dreams were alleviated. She also reported general relief from her muscle aches and pains.

While auricular acupuncture is an appropriate and important component of any substance abuse treatment program, it is by no means the only component. A patient's behavior and attitude, along with the perceptions of the clinician delivering care, are also integral to successful treatment. Although extremely effective, it is a complementary approach to treatment and recovery support groups. Substance abuse treatment must address the whole person. It is vital that the person learn new and effective coping skills to deal with the stressors in their life. They must learn to socialize and celebrate without the use of mind-altering substances. In many cases, they need to address patterns of behavior that have created pain and suffering in their lives. Healthy boundaries must be learned and maintained. In some cases, the person needs to learn healthy eating and wellness habits. Above all, the person must have an improvement in their self-image. It is my experience that people with healthy self-esteem will cease self-destructive behavior.

Auricular acupuncture is a viable component in the treatment of addiction, anxiety, depression, and stress-related disorders. The greatest benefit is the ability of acupuncture to relieve the discomfort of withdrawal, and to address the anxiety and depression often present in the first few months of recovery with limited use or without the use of psychotropic medications. The use of acupuncture helps the recovering person manage cravings, reducing the likelihood of relapse. This wonderful complementary protocol helps the client become better engaged in the treatment process and remain in treatment longer, greatly improving treatment outcomes. Studies have shown that the longer a person is engaged in treatment, the more successful they will be in their efforts for long-term recovery.

14

Is Relapse a Necessary Part of Recovery?

"We keep moving forward, opening new doors, and doing new things, because we're curious and curiosity keeps leading us down new paths."
—Walt Disney

What is a relapse? A relapse is a breakdown or setback in one's attempts to change or modify any target behavior. A relapse can manifest itself in a progressive pattern of behavior that reactivates the symptoms of the disease. These symptoms could show themselves as:

- Irritability
- Obsessive, compulsive thoughts and behavior
- Feelings of discontent
- Interruption of sleep patterns
- High levels of frustration
- Anxiety

- Unusual outbursts

An important component of recovery is to become aware of your feelings and corresponding behaviors. When people are active in an addiction, they are not always in touch with their emotions. In fact, addicts are using their drug or behavior of choice to avoid feelings. In learning the relapse cycle and identifying how we relate to each component of it, we learn to differentiate emotions, thoughts, and actions. This helps us learn to act instead of react. One of the positive aspects of recovery is that we are forced to know ourselves in a very real way.

When people relapse, it is usually when they are faced with a high-risk situation and are not prepared for it. High-risk situations include:

- The loss of a job
- The death of a friend or loved one
- A divorce
- Running into old "using" buddies
- Children leaving home
- Depression
- Physical, mental, or emotional illness
- Complacency

Some people may self-sabotage recovery due to lack of coping skills, self-esteem, or lack of preparation. One of my most important goals in developing this program and for writing this book has been to give recovering people self-empowering tools that last a lifetime.

> I've had the joy of watching many people as they heal from the effects of addiction, rediscover themselves; and enjoy full, emotionally rich, and healthy lifestyles.

Health and wellness must address all parts of people's lives. They need the tools to understand physical fitness and nutrition, emotional and mental health, and healthy social interactions. They need support that encourages sobriety, enjoyment, spiritual growth, and development. Living well takes commitment in all of these areas.

The methods I have offered have reaped tremendous progress in the lives of the individuals I have worked with. I've had the joy of watching many people as they heal from the effects of addiction, rediscover themselves; and enjoy full, emotionally rich, and healthy lifestyles.

I have heard it said that relapse is just part of the process, and sometimes it is. But people do not have to relapse. Success can and does happen. In addition to learning the life skills discussed so far, I use a system of relapse prevention with my clients that is simple, to the point, and works well.

Relapse does not begin with the use of the drug. Relapse begins with a trigger and the emotions surrounding it. Feelings arise from the way we perceive things and the thoughts we have as a result. Unlike thoughts, our feelings create a physical reaction in our bodies. Some of our feelings may be at the surface, and others may be suppressed.

We cannot think away the feelings we have surrounding an area of our lives, but we can reduce the unnecessary and unfounded self-blame, guilt, and shame by learning to distinguish between self-blame and personal responsibility. Self-blame and guilt can trigger relapse. Self-blame arises in part because powerlessness and helplessness are two of the worst feelings a human can experience. Therefore, people often blame themselves for negative events in order to feel that they are in control. Self-blame is different than taking personal responsibility for our lives. Self-blame is self-deprecating and leads to deeper shame. Taking responsibility acknowledges that we have made choices in our lives that have negative results, and that we are willing to grow from those mistakes. Taking responsibility gives us the option of seeing the lessons we've learned and seizing the opportunities to grow as individuals.

Relapse always follows a pattern, and if we learn what is happening within us, we can learn to avoid that painful pattern. Keep in mind that the healthier we are physically, emotionally, mentally, and spiritually, the more easily behaviors and thoughts that do not serve us well will fall away. I am not saying that triggers won't happen. It is just that when they do, they will have little or no power over us.

Let's look at each step of this cycle. It always begins with a trigger. A trigger can be anything, such as thoughts, signs, smells, people; or situations that cause us to want to drink; use drugs; or reengage in self-destructive behavior.

I have used this model for many years, and I have never had anyone who was not able to identify with it. The pattern looks like this:

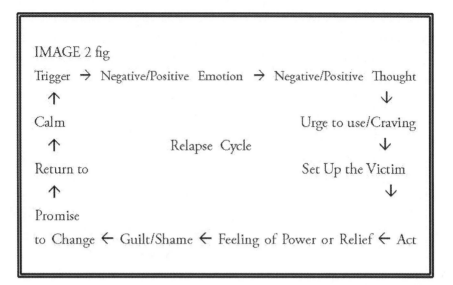

IMAGE 2 fig

Trigger → Negative/Positive Emotion → Negative/Positive Thought

↑ ↓

Calm   Urge to use/Craving

↑   Relapse Cycle   ↓

Return to   Set Up the Victim

↑   ↓

Promise

to Change ← Guilt/Shame ← Feeling of Power or Relief ← Act

Following the trigger, we experience negative emotions, such as frustration, restlessness, anxiety, stress, or anger. Interestingly, triggers can also be positive emotions, such as excitement or a feeling of accomplishment; in this case, the trigger is not followed by negative emotions. Whether experienced negatively or positively, however, triggers are always followed by negative thoughts. A negative thought in this context would be something like:

- *I deserve a drink.*
- *"One or two won't hurt anything."*
- *"I can handle it."*
- *"I'm tired of this recovery thing!"*
- *"Forget it—who cares?"*

At this point, people no longer consider the consequences of relapse, or if they do, they begin to minimize the consequences. This is when our "self-will" sets in; we think, *"I want what I want, when I want it, and I don't care who gets in the way, I am going to get it."*

What follows is an urge to use or to participate in addictive behavior—in other words, a craving. Cravings are strong desires that, if not intervened on, will lead to relapse.

Intervention can come from the recovering addicts themselves. Coping strategies include redirecting our thinking and getting busy. I teach my clients the "3-3-3 rule": when you experience a trigger to fall back into old behavior, you have three seconds to redirect your thoughts. If three seconds don't work, give yourself three minutes, then three hours. This works well if you're emotional, upset, or angry. It is amazing how differently we see a situation if we separate from it for three hours!

Practice some deep breathing, Pray, consider the positive aspects of your recovery, and call your sponsor or someone who understands and who will talk you through it. Go to a meeting; be around sober people who are interested in your and their own well-being. Remember, positive energy creates positive energy. Negative energy creates negative energy. Take care of yourself. You are worth it.

If you can, practice some yoga poses. By leaning into the pose slowly, then changing positions slowly, you can change your perspective. Practice chakra balancing; it can help to align your energy and get out of the anxiousness that cravings bring about. Give yourself a few minutes to close your eyes and focus on each energy field. You will be amazed at how much better you feel.

Above all, this is not the time to call your dealer or drug-using friends!

Following the urge to use, people "set up the victim." The victim here is the addict who relapses. Setting up the victim is the ritual of calling, looking for, and obtaining the drug. It may mean stopping by the bar "just to say hi." Setting up the victim may mean calling the person we have an addiction to, "just to find closure," or "just to make sure they're okay." Remember, it isn't about them—it is about you, and feeding your addiction.

After we set up the victim comes the *act*. The act is drinking, using, or returning to old behaviors. Keep in mind that there have been five steps prior to this point—and when we are aware of what is happening, we can intervene anywhere along the way. It isn't always easy, but we'll feel better about ourselves if we do.

As soon as people have a drink, a smoke, a hit, or whatever, they experience an immediate feeling of relief, even power. This may last for a little while—but it soon goes away, and the problems caused by addiction remain or become even worse.

When we go against our commitments to ourselves and other people, we usually feel a sense of shame or guilt, especially if we know that the behavior is wrong, illegal, or will cause relationship problems. This is the core of addiction—and it often keeps the vicious cycle going. People then use in order to relieve the feelings of guilt, creating an even bigger problem.

After the drama of relapse comes the promise to reform. Phrases such as "I'm sorry," "I'll never do it again," "I love you," and "Don't leave me," are common. At the time that people are sick, hung over, or in trouble, they honestly mean it. The loved ones—or the legal system—however, doubt addicts' sincerity. After all, this is not the first time they have heard these words from addicts.

Now things begin to return to calm. There is still mistrust and hurt, but typically both people want things to be better. This is sometimes called "the honeymoon period." The addict is feeling better and treating people with kindness and respect—and is possibly doing things to get back in everyone's good graces. Everyone, including the addict, hopes that this time is the real deal.

Relapse hurts everyone, most especially addicts. Relapse does not have to happen, although sometimes it does. If addicts approach a relapse with a true desire to understand what happened—and to grow and continue to make changes—they can move past and learn from it. If a relapse should happen, it is imperative that addicts continue to work on their programs of recovery. We *can* break free from the cycle!

Remember that recovery is about self-discovery. It is about establishing good boundaries and making decisions that create growth and positive outcomes in our lives. It is about gaining and re-establishing our personal dignity and self-respect.

Addiction is a lifestyle, and so is sobriety. When we choose sobriety, we must redefine our lifestyles. It is not always easy, for there will be people who we love and care for who will continue on the path of addiction. Sometimes, we must leave them behind. Sometimes, we will question if we have made the right choice, especially if it appears that those we left behind are having a good time, and we are feeling left out.

It's said that when we are addicted, we are playing with a rattlesnake without realizing it is a rattlesnake. When we're on the road to recovery, we see that it is a rattlesnake and we play with it anyway, thinking that we won't get hurt. When we become healthy and we see a rattlesnake, we walk on the other side of the path. This makes good sense to me.

I would like to encourage the reader to avoid focusing on the possibility of relapse; it's more important to focus on a healthy, balanced lifestyle. To maintain emotional health and to minimize triggers, we must learn to focus on what we *do* want, not on what we don't want, including relapse. I will repeat this important thought once more: whatever we focus on, we create in our lives. We must learn to live in today. To do this, we look at the past and the lessons learned, and then let it go. We don't dwell there. Focusing on the past can keep old triggers alive and kicking. In contrast, getting in touch with your creativity and your passions can help you live your life to the fullest.

That said, understand that once your brain has become addicted, it will always remember and maximize the pleasure sensation and deny or minimize the negative consequences. Any use of the substance will create cravings that will not allow addicted people to use moderately. The addicted brain has no stop sign!

My deepest desire is for you to love yourself and live your life well. Understand your goodness. Never doubt your ability to be happy, joyous, and free. Living a life of integrity, which means being whole, is the greatest gift you can give yourself.

Conclusion

Recovery is not a destination. It is a journey that those of us with addictions must take. As I discussed in chapter three, we were *not* born in a broken, imperfect state. We were born perfect, even if that perfection doesn't meet someone else's definition of perfection. When a baby is born, they are in their most honest, pure state. When they feel an emotion, they feel it all over. Imagine a baby laughing. They laugh all over! Imagine a baby who's angry because she isn't being fed fast enough to suit her. Is there any doubt about what she's feeling?

It is through life experiences that we develop defenses, complexes, and beliefs that define us as bad; not good enough; not smart enough; or less than others. In order to deal with our perceived imperfections, we develop coping mechanisms to help us along. The lower our self-esteem, the more self-defeating these coping mechanisms become. The more we disapprove of ourselves, the more we disapprove of others. The more dishonoring we are to ourselves, the more dishonoring we will be to others.

It is through the process of recovery that we become whole again. In Christianity, this can be viewed as the process of salvation; as dying to ourselves and being born again through Christ. In Eastern philosophy, this can be understood as the way of enlightenment or awakening. Either way we see it, we are brought back to a place of unity with our highest self. This may be called God, Christ-consciousness, a state of bliss, or nirvana.

Belief systems that are driven by fear, shame, and guilt are what lead us into addictions and self-destructive behaviors. This book is about healing. It is about drawing on tools from many disciplines in order to live a life of wholeness and health.

Western allopathic medications can have a place in healing from addiction; they can help alleviate the pain of withdrawal and balance brain chemistry negatively affected by the environment, overstimulation, or drug abuse. Western medicine has come far in helping people manage or heal from life-threatening illnesses. However, it has also enabled people to alleviate symptoms without addressing underlying problems. The symptoms return and the problems repeat over and over again, often defining and controlling people's lives.

The Twelve Step program of Alcoholics Anonymous also has a place in recovery; it gives us a sober, social support system and a path for developing accountability and personal integrity. Some people have said that AA and the Twelve Steps have returned them to sanity after the hopelessness and insanity of addiction. It does, however, keep us dependent on the program and does not empower us to heal ourselves through coping tools. A basic principle of AA is that once people are "sick" with the disease of addiction, they are doomed to struggle with it for the rest of their lives. It fosters the idea of remission versus the idea of healing and wholeness.

The holistic approach to recovery addresses the whole person. It encourages people to embrace health and wellness in all its aspects. Physical health is addressed through diet, exercise, and deep, conscious breathing; spiritual and emotional health are addressed through prayer, meditation,, and positive affirmation; mental health is addressed through guided imagery, personal growth, and self-discipline; and social health is addressed through the ideas of respect of self, others, and the environment. That said, what the holistic approach lacks is the social support of AA.

Each of these methodologies has its strengths and weaknesses. Together, they form a dynamic approach to helping us achieve wholeness in all areas of our lives. This complementary approach to recovery gives us the tools to return to a life of peace, power, and a sound mind.

Bibliography

The Big Book of Alcoholics Anonymous. 4th ed., New York: Alcoholics Anonymous World Service, 2002.

The Big Book of Alcoholics Anonymous. 3rd ed., New York: Alcoholics Anonymous World Service, 1976.

Harris, Bill. *Thresholds of the Mind.* Beaverton, OR: Centerpointe Research Institute, 2007.

Hendricks, Gay. *Conscious Breathing.* New York: Bantam Books, 1995.

Howard, Pierce J. *The Owner's Manual for the Brain.* Austin, TX: Bard Press, 2004.

Lee, Ilchi. *Brain Wave Vibration.* Sedona, AZ: Best Life Media, 2008.

Letts, Pamela J., Philip R. A. Baker, James Ruderman, and Kennedy Karen. "The Use of Hypnosis in Labor and Delivery: A Preliminary Study." *Journal of Women's Health* 2, no. 4 (1993): 335–341.

Miller, Emmett E. *Deep Healing.* Carlsbad, CA: Hay House, 2008.

Pinkola Estés, Clarissa. *Women Who Run with the Wolves.* New York: Ballantine Books, 1992.

Rinpoche, Sogyal. *The Tibetan Book of Living and Dying.* New York: HarperCollins, 1994.

Sherwood, Keith. *Chakra Therapy.* St. Paul, MN: Llewelynn, 2002.

Sturgess, Stephen. *The Yoga Book.* London: Watkins, 2002.